BLUEPRINT
FOR
GRID-DOWN
SURVIVAL

Power up Your Readiness with Expert
Tips, Tactical Hacks, Essential First Aid,
CPR, and Comprehensive Checklists

NORKOR OMABOE

CONTENTS

FROM THE SAME AUTHOR

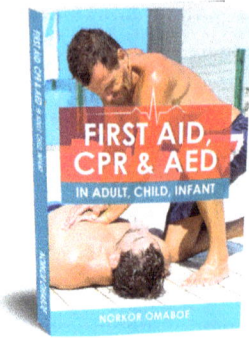

First Aid, CPR & AED: In Adult, Child, Infant by Norkor Omaboe

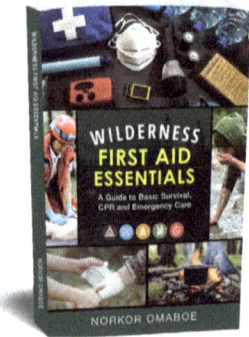

Wilderness First Aid Essentials: A Guide to Survival, CPR, and Emergency Care by Norkor Omaboe

INTRODUCTION

Disasters are becoming more common, and with them, the need to be prepared. Many experts point to climate change as a major factor in the rise of extreme weather events, but it is not just about the weather. Cyberattacks, pandemics, and civil unrest are some of the many possible threats that can disrupt our way of life. And... we are left with no communication, no water, and mainly, no electricity. But a true grid down situation is far more serious implications that most of us can realize.

For most people, the gravity of the situation may not sink in until after a few days without water or electricity. When uncertain times breed uncertainty, does it mean we should continue living in fear? Not at all. Rather than waiting, how do you recognize that it is indeed a grid down? You can step ahead and prepare so you stay in control before the general panic. But the question is, how?

Blueprint for Grid-Down Survival is your ultimate guide to not only survive but thrive in a grid-down situation. Here is a breakdown of what you will find inside:

- How to be prepared for limited or zero power

- Practical tips and strategies to thrive through a power outage with confidence

- Urban survival tactics to keep you safe in a city environment

- Creative cooking solutions without relying on electric appliances

- Sourcing and purifying water in an urban setting

- Maintaining communication during an emergency

- Essential first aid for adults, and infants

There's an old saying: *Si vis pacem, para bellum*, that translates to, *If you want peace, prepare for war.* It might sound strange, but it basically means this: Hope for the best but plan for the worst (Roberts, 2023). This guide is all about that second part: being prepared for a situation where the power goes out for a long time. By planning ahead, you can make sure you and your family are safe and comfortable even when things get tough.

Start slow, but start today!

1

UNVEILING URBAN PERILS—IDENTIFYING IMPENDING GRID-DOWN CRISES

You are glued to the screen, desperate to know who the killer is in your favorite show. Just when the scene is about to reveal the real culprit, Bam! Darkness. The power is out. You check your phone: no signal. You walk outside your house: no street lights. You go back inside, turn the faucet on: no water. Within a few days, the food in your fridge starts to spoil, grocery stores are empty; within a week or so, sewage overflow, and general panic arise. The first question that comes to mind is: What is causing this?

In this chapter, let's discover the possible causes that can result in a grid-down situation.

LEARNING OBJECTIVES

After reading this chapter, you will be able to:

- Understand different scenarios that can lead to a long-term grid-down

- Report and track a grid-down in your area

- Analyze the consequences of an urban grid-down

IDENTIFYING POTENTIAL TRIGGERS FOR GRID-DOWN SCENARIOS

While a complete power outage might sound like something out of a dystopian movie, the reality is that grid-down scenarios are a genuine possibility. Here's why:

NATURAL DISASTERS

Recent years have been a wake-up call when it comes to power outages caused by natural disasters. Hurricane Sandy, the Japan Earthquake, and Hurricane Katrina all resulted in long-term grid-downs. These are just a few examples, and the situation is only expected to get worse. The reason is simple: Climate change is amplifying both the frequency and intensity of natural disasters.

Some common natural disasters that can cause grid-down situations include hurricanes, tropical storms, earthquakes, tornadoes, wildfires, floods, volcanic eruptions, and landslides.

CYBERATTACKS

While a physical attack with bombs or missiles might be the first thing that comes to mind, cyber threats have become a growing concern for power grids around the world. Cyberattacks can range from data theft to system disruption, with the potential to cause widespread blackouts.

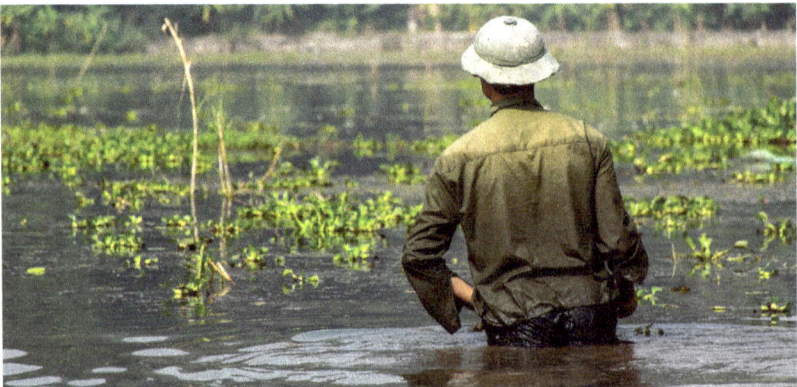

Did you know that 86.8% of power outages are caused by natural disasters? (*The Impact of Power Outages*, n.d.).

EQUIPMENT FAILURE

Over time, electrical components like transformers, cables, and circuit breakers can wear down or malfunction. This can lead to overheating, short circuits, or complete breakdowns. Even properly maintained equipment can fail due to unexpected surges or manufacturing defects. When this happens, safety systems may automatically shut down the flow of electricity to prevent damage, resulting in a blackout.

Info-Bite
A *blackout* is "a complete loss of power in a specific area that results in no electricity for a long period of time," whereas a *brownout* is "a partial, temporary reduction in voltage from the power supply that causes the lights to dim."

HOW TO TRACK A GRID-DOWN?

You can stay informed about the status of a grid-down by tracking the scope of the problem through various channels. Here's how you can do it:

CONSIDER OUTAGE MAPS

Most utility companies maintain online outage maps accessible through their websites or mobile apps. These real-time maps provide visual confirmation of outages in your neighborhood and will allow you to see the extent of the problem.

Refer to the Outage Information Pages
By clicking on the outage icon on the map, a user is usually directed to a dedicated "Outage Information" page. This page provides important details such as the following:

- The estimated restoration time gives an idea of when to expect the power to be back on.

- The time reported represents the time when the first outage report was made.

- The cause of the outage.

- The status of restoration provides insight into the ongoing repair work and any updates from the utility company.

These resources are constantly updated, so it is best to check back periodically to get new information.

CONSEQUENCES OF A POWER GRID-DOWN

Our world runs on electricity. Thus, a long-term grid failure can disturb everything from our basic needs to even the fabric of our society. Without electricity, food supplies go short, communication becomes challenging, basic needs like clean water and sanitation are compromised, and economic activities come to a pause. These conditions can lead to widespread panic, looting, and a breakdown of essential services.

While it might sound daunting, there are steps you can take to increase your chances of staying safe and comfortable throughout a grid-down scenario. There are three pillars of urban survival in a long-term power outage (*Urban Survival Training*, n.d.):

- **Preparation is power:** This is your first line of defense. Stock essential supplies like food, water, and first aid items to meet your basic needs. Have an action plan for your family ready.

- **Resourcefulness is key:** You will need to be resourceful and use what's available in your surroundings. Think beyond your pantry and explore different options to cook without electricity.

- **Mindset matters most:** Stay calm, focused, and adaptable to make sound decisions and cope with stress.

TO SUM UP

So, we have talked about the triggers of a grid-down, along with some consequences so far. But are *you* prepared? Take a quick quiz!

- Think of three disasters that can cause long-term grid-downs.

- Can you tell the difference between a blackout and a brownout?—hint: one dims, the other disappears!

CHAPTER 2

IMMEDIATE CRISIS MANAGEMENT— TACTICAL SOLUTIONS FOR URBAN RESILIENCE

As soon as the power goes out, your cozy home might start feeling scary in the shadows. But just before you start picturing monsters under the bed, take a deep breath. This chapter is your battle plan to survive the first few moments of a grid-down. It aims to equip you with the knowledge and skills to come out of the initial chaos feeling strong and capable.

LEARNING OBJECTIVES

By the end of this chapter, you will be able to:

- Learn effective strategies to manage the initial surge of panic and anxiety

- Develop a clear action plan to prioritize immediate safety needs for yourself and your loved ones

- 3-Day Action Plan Sample

MAINTAINING CALM AND ORDER IN THE INITIAL MOMENTS

In a grid-down scenario, staying calm is important to make clear, rational decisions. Learning basic relaxation skills can be useful in any stressful situation. Here is how to stay ahead of the panic and take charge:

TRY THE BOX BREATHING TECHNIQUE

The Box Breathing technique is used by the Navy Seals to quickly calm the nervous system in high stress situations. It is easy to learn and can help clear your mind of racing thoughts and bring your attention back to the present moment. A quick way to de-stress and refocus is box breathing. Ready to give it a try? Here's how:

1. Breathe in slowly through your nose for four seconds. Feel your belly and chest expand as your lungs fill with air.

2. Pause for four seconds without inhaling and exhaling.

3. Slowly release the air through your mouth for four seconds. Now, feel your belly and chest sink back to their normal position.

4. Hold your breath for another four seconds.

5. Continue repeating these steps for several cycles until you feel a sense of calm wash over you.

ACKNOWLEDGE YOUR FEELINGS

It is okay to feel scared or overwhelmed in this situation. Don't judge yourself for those emotions, but don't let them control you, either. Here is how you can validate your emotions:

- Verbally talk out your feelings to process your emotions and reduce the intensity. Say things like, "This is scary," or, "I feel overwhelmed right now."

- While you acknowledge the fear, challenge any negative thoughts that may arise. For instance, instead of thinking, *I am going to be stuck like this forever*, tell yourself, "This is temporary, and I can take steps to cope."

- Shift your focus from the problem to potential solutions. Ask yourself, "What can I do right now to feel more prepared?" This will help you take your mind off the anxiety.

KEEP OTHERS CALM
Confidence is contagious. Stay composed and speak in a reassuring tone. This will help ease the nervousness of your family and neighbors.

AVOID SPREADING MISINFORMATION
Misinformation or assumptions can quickly increase the panic. Therefore, make sure to remember these pointers when sharing information with family or neighbors:

- Only share verified information from trusted sources like official broadcasts or local authorities.

- Avoid spreading rumors or speculation.

- Highlight the resources available.

- Avoid using technical terms and focus on delivering information in a way everyone can understand.

TAKING CHARGE AND DELEGATING TASKS

In order to keep things running smoothly within your household, take charge and develop an action. This will look different for every family, but the basics remain the same.

Start by getting a quick head count and understanding everyone's specific needs. Depending on the ability of each person, delegate tasks. Here's a sneak peek into how:

- When assigning tasks, consider individual strengths and abilities. For instance, someone with medical knowledge could be responsible for administering medications, while a handy person could focus on securing the house. It is best to determine roles before the crisis as well.

- Keep it simple and specific while delegating. Clearly explain each task and the desired outcome.

- Let everyone know you trust their abilities. Offer encouragement and praise for a job well done.

Tasks that require delegation include an immediate hazard check, exterior and interior safety check (closing windows, locking doors, or investigating any tripping hazards), information gathering, flashlight distribution, and first aid check—attending to the medical needs based on the situation.

ASSESSING THE SITUATION

Run an immediate safety check. Look out for any potential hazards that might be a contributing cause to the situation.

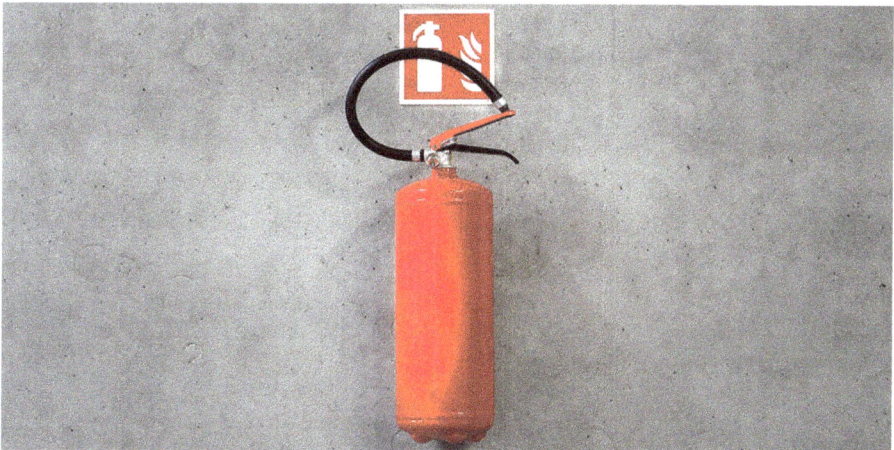

TAKE A QUICK VISUAL CHECK FOR IMMEDIATE DANGERS

A quick visual check allows you to identify and address immediate safety concerns before anyone gets injured. This could
mean extinguishing potential fire hazards or clearing tripping
hazards before people start moving around in the dark.

Hazard	Indicator	What to do
Fire	Flames, smoke, or a burning smell.	1. *Evacuate immediately.* Ensure everyone in the vicinity of the fire is aware and moving toward safety. 2. *Call your local emergency number* to notify firefighters of the fire. 3. Once outside, stay there. Reentering a burning building puts you at risk of smoke inhalation, structural collapse, or becoming trapped.
Gas leakage	Sulfur-like odor or a scent similar to rotten eggs.	• If you know where the gas meter is and can safely access it, *turn off the gas supply*. The valve is typically turned a quarter turn—90°—so that it is perpendicular to the pipe to shut off the gas.

- *Do not use matches, lighters, or any electrical devices*—including light switches and phones—inside the building.

- *Move at least 300 ft—100 m—away* from the building to ensure your safety in case of an explosion.

| Noise from appliances | Unusual sounds such as buzzing, clicking, or hissing, coming from electrical appliances. | 4. If safe to do so, *immediately turn off the appliance* and unplug it from the power source. 5. Carefully inspect the appliance for any visible signs of damage, such as frayed cords, burnt marks, or loose parts. 6. *Contact a qualified appliance repair technician* to diagnose and fix the issue. Avoid using the appliance until it has been inspected and repaired. |

Unusual odors	Any strange or unfamiliar smells, especially those resembling burning rubber or chemicals, can indicate a serious problem.	• Try to *locate the source of the smell* if it's safe to do so. This could be an electrical appliance, chemical spill, or other potential hazard. • *Open windows and doors* to allow fresh air to circulate and ventilate the space.

IDENTIFY SAFE AND UNSAFE AREAS AROUND YOU

If the grid-down is a result of a disaster, you must know where to go. Here is how to assess your surroundings and identify areas that are safe and unsafe during emergencies:

Shelter-In-Place

Shelter-in-place means "finding a safe room inside a building and staying there until it is safe to leave. It is ideal when outside conditions pose a greater threat than staying indoors."

Who decides that? Local authorities may issue a shelter-in-place order during emergencies like:

- Criminal activity—active shooter, armed individuals

- Natural disasters—tornadoes, hailstorms, heavy snow

- Hazardous material release—chemical, biological, radiological

Evacuation

Blaring sirens can send shivers down anyone's spine. But in the heat of the moment, if authorities issue a mandatory evacuation order, leave immediately. Do not wait to see how the situation unfolds.

Some situations demand immediate evacuation, regardless of official orders. These include:

- Flooding

- Fire

- Gas leaks

- Downed power lines

Making the Right Call
When assessing the situation, you need to make the right call between staying at your home, choosing a shelter-in-place, or evacuating immediately.

If you suspect any immediate dangers or authorities is-sue an evacuation order, prioritize leaving the area for a safe location. When immediate threats are absent and sheltering indoors might be preferable, look for an interior room without windows or one that can be effectively sealed off for maximum protection.

STAYING SAFE THROUGH ALL

Prevention is key to staying safe during a power outage. Prioritize safety by taking the following actions:

- Secure your home. Locate and familiarize yourself with gas, water, and electrical shutoff points. Turn them off during a power outage to prevent damage when the power returns. Only turn off gas valves if you suspect a leak and know how to do it safely.

- Create safe zones by choosing an interior room away from windows and exterior walls. Stock it with essen-tials like blankets, flashlights, a radio, a first aid kit, and supplies. Read more on creating a ready-to-go bag packed with all the necessary items in Chapter 5. Make sure to keep a fire extinguisher near your safe zone for easy access.

ESTABLISHING A COMMUNICATION PLAN

In a grid-down scenario, traditional communication methods may fail, so it is important to have a plan in place. To establish a communication plan:

- Create a physical notebook with important contact information as a reliable backup to electronic devices such as a mobile phone.

- Engage with your neighbors to establish a support system, share resources, and organize community patrols to enhance safety.

- Prioritize the well-being of vulnerable individuals and set up a system for reporting suspicious activity to maintain security and community support.

STAYING INFORMED

Don't be left in the dark—literally and figuratively! Make frequent information checks a priority during a grid-down. Here are some tips:

- Battery-powered or hand-crank emergency radios are your best bet for reliable updates during a power outage. Tune in to local emergency broadcasts for official information about the outage, safety instructions, and estimated restoration times.

- Check in with your local TDSP if the outage's reason is unknown. They can provide updates on the outage's cause, scope, and estimated restoration time.

- If you have some cell service or can connect to Wi-Fi at a community hotspot, use the official apps from local authorities or trusted news organizations. These apps can provide real-time updates and important safety information. However, do not forget to prioritize battery life and avoid draining your phone unnecessarily.

During a grid-down, local authorities become your primary source of guidance. Pay close attention to their instructions and follow any safety protocols they advise. This could include evacuation orders, boil water notices, or curfews.

GRID DOWN ACTION PLAN
Day 1
- Delegate

- Locate all family members and pets and get everyone home

- Find out the likely cause of the grid-down. Set up camp stove, grill or pit

- Collect water

- Purchase emergency lighting:

  o Flashlights, headlights, hurricane and batteries and battery operated radio

  o Hurricane lanterns (they stay lit even with strong winds)

  o Propane lanterns (they generate heat but should only be used in well ventilated area)

  o LED lanterns can lit a whole room and are energy efficient. However you will need to stock on batteries

- Create a list of food items that can last without spoiling when there is no electricity
- Establish lighting with candles, oil lamps, LED lamps and flash lights
- Set up a no electricity kitchen
- Set up alternative cooking equipment
- Create an inventory of resources. Plan meals to minimize waste.
- Assess nearby water sources
- Go grocery shopping if it is safe to do so

Day 2
- Disconnect your property from public utilities
- Start purifying water
- Hygiene: set up a waste disposal system

Day 3
- Secure your property,
- Connect with neighbors to determine if collaboration is beneficial and safe. Share updates with trusted neighbors.
- Develop a system of night watch.
- Prepare for possible evacuation

TO SUM UP

To turn the initial chaos of a grid-down into control, a proactive approach is key. By taking immediate steps to secure your environment, establish communication channels, and create a plan of action, you can get through this situation. You have got this!

3

CULINARY INGENUITY—COOKING STRATEGIES FOR URBAN SURVIVAL

So, no microwave, no air fryer, no oven, no cooktop, no slow cooker, and no blender. Then, what? There are plenty of options available when it comes to cooking off-grid. Let's take a look at both outdoor and indoor options for you to choose from.

LEARNING OBJECTIVES

In this chapter, we'll be looking at the following:

- Alternative cooking methods, both indoors and outdoors
- Tips for stocking up in advance
- Nutrition requirements when using alternative food sources and cooking methods

INDOOR COOKING METHODS

Indoor cooking during a grid-down requires extra care. Limited space in the kitchen means fires and smoke spread quicker than outdoors. Therefore, prioritize ventilation, keep the windows and doors open, or set up near a window or balcony. Most importantly, have a fire extinguisher ready at all times!

"CAQUELON"

A *caquelon*—pronounced *kah-kə-lon*—is "a traditional pot typically used for preparing fondue." But its uses extend far beyond cheese! Made from durable materials like stoneware, ceramic, enameled cast iron, or porcelain, a caquelon can be a valuable addition to your kitchen for a grid-down. Here's how:

- You can use it over a camp stove or portable burner to boil water, simmer soup and stews, or even cook rice.

- Sauté vegetables, simmer sauces, or heat precooked meals as caquelon's versatility makes it a resourceful cooking tool.

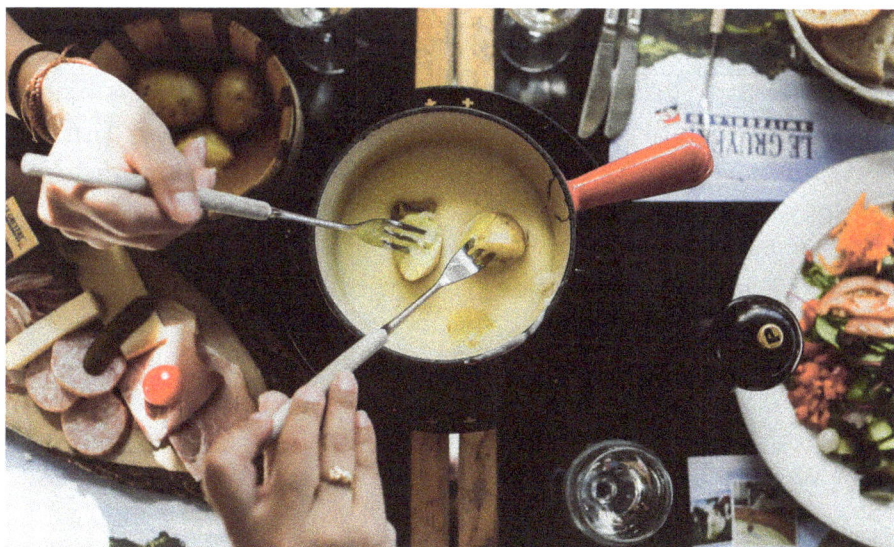

Required Tools
- *Caquelon.* They often come as a set and include the gelled fuel or gel alcohol to heat the food. Ensure you purchase extra gelled fuel.

- Heat source—camp stove, portable burner

- Utensils for cooking—spoons, spatula

How to Use a Caquelon?
1. Place your *caquelon* on a stable heat source like a camp stove, a portable burner or the gelled fuel.

2. Add your desired ingredients—water for boiling, vegetables for soup, etc.—and cook according to your recipe.

Tips
- Enameled cast iron *caquelons* retain heat well. Use low heat to avoid burning your food.

- Once cool, wash your *caquelon* with warm, soapy water.

OUTDOOR COOKING METHODS

Open fires and grills offer a wider range of cooking possibilities compared to limited indoor options during a power outage. You can roast, boil, smoke, and even bake with some outdoor setups.

Here are the best outdoor cooking options to explore:

CAMPFIRE COOKING

Campfire cooking doesn't have to be all hot dogs and marshmallows. Simmer stews, sear meats for smoky goodness, roast veggies in foil, and even bake in a Dutch oven!

Required Tools
- Firewood

- Lighter

- Grill grate

- Cast iron

- Dutch oven

- Aluminum foil

- Water–dirt

How to Set a Campfire?
- Build your fire pit in a clear area, away from flammable objects like tents, trees, or bushes. Surround it with rocks to create a contained cooking space.

- You will need a variety of firewood sizes. Dry, seasoned wood is essential for a clean and hot fire. Small kindling for starting, finger-sized sticks for building the fire, and larger logs for long-term burning will suit you.

- Use a grill grate over the fire.

- Knowing when to use direct and indirect heat is the key to campfire cooking success. Direct heat—cooking directly over the flames—is ideal for searing and quick cooking. Indirect heat—placing your pan near the edge of the fire—is perfect for simmering, stewing, or baking.

- Usually, a campfire can be put off by pouring plenty of water onto the embers and coals. If water is scarce due to a grid-down, you can carefully use dirt to smother the embers. Similar to water, completely cover the embers and ash with a thick layer of dirt, then stir it up to ensure everything is extinguished.

Safety Tips
- Never leave a fire unattended.

- Keep a bucket of water or sand–dirt nearby to extinguish the fire if needed.

- Do not burn trash or anything other than clean, dry firewood.

GRILL

Grilling is a fantastic way to cook delicious food outdoors. You can choose between using charcoal or propane based on your personal preference and cooking experience.

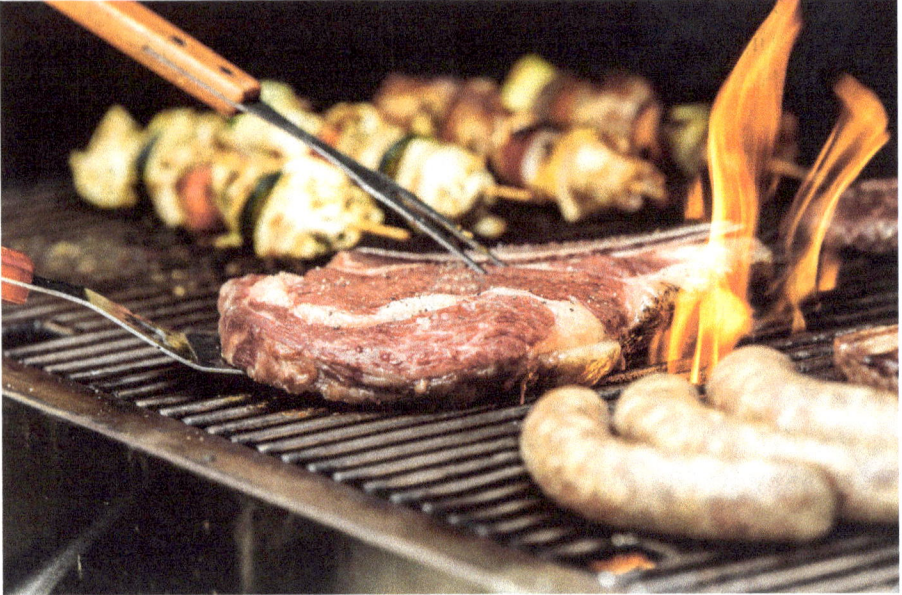

Required Tools
- grill, of course
- fuel (propane–charcoal briquette)
- tongs
- instant-read digital thermometer

Note
Charcoal grills deliver a smoky flavor and high heat, which is good when it comes to searing, but require lighting and involve more cleanup. Propane grills, on the other hand, offer instant on, precise temperature control, and easier cleaning, but you will have to drop the smoky taste.

How to Use a Grill?

1. Make sure that you have enough charcoal or a full pro-pane tank. If you are opting for charcoal, you will have to decide between briquettes—slower burn—or lump charcoal—faster burn)

2. Start with a clean grill for even cooking and preventing flare-ups.

3. Light charcoal or turn the propane knob on to ignite. Preheat to medium-high.

4. If you are on charcoal, open the bottom vent fully. Unlike propane grills, this vent controls airflow and heat in a charcoal grill. A fully open vent allows optimal oxygen for the fire. Conversely, propane grills have knobs for ignition and heat control.

5. Grill your food and enjoy.

Tips to Use a Grill

• Scrub grates for a clean cooking surface and lightly oil to prevent sticking.

• Set up a side table for cooked food, seasoning, and utensils.

• Always check the internal temperatures of meat with a digital thermometer for safe consumption.

FUELING THE FIRE

Stocking up on the fire fuel is critical and depends on the cook-ing methods. Knowledge is key to understand what makes most sense in your situation.

• Matches

• Lighter fluids

- Fire starter tablets

- Coal

- Pre-cut resin rich wood

- Gel fuel

SOLAR OVEN

Skip the fire and use the power of the sun. The easiest solution is to purchase a solar oven. A solar cooker can help you heat, cook, and even pasteurize your food and drinks. Alternatively, you can make a DIY style solar oven.

Required Tools
- Cardboard box

- Aluminum foil

- Clear plastic wrap

- Black construction paper

- Ruler

- Glue stick

- Tape

- Stick for propping the lid open

- Scissors

How to DIY a Solar Oven?
1. With the help of a ruler and box cutter, carefully cut a three-sided flap on the top of a box lid. Leave about 1 in. of border around the edges. You want this flap to fold up and become a reflector.

2. Line the inside of the flap you just cut with aluminum foil. You can use glue to secure it for a smoother finish. This will reflect sunlight into the box.

3. Cut a similar-sized opening on the opposite side of the box lid. This will be your window. Cover this opening with clear plastic wrap or an oven bag, and seal it tightly with tape to create an airtight window.

4. Line the inside bottom of the cardboard box with black construction paper or paint it black. Black absorbs heat efficiently, and this will be the cooking surface where you will place your food.

5. Once everything is dry, fold the reflector flap you created. Prop the lid open with your stick at an angle that directs sunlight into the window and onto the black bottom.

Tips

- Aim the oven directly at the sun and adjust the angle throughout the day to maximize heat collection.

- Insulate the box with cardboard scraps or towels for better heat retention.

- Solar ovens are great for slow cooking. Think stews, casseroles, or baked goods.

- Preheat your oven for 20–30 minutes before adding food.

- Use dark-colored pots for better heat absorption.

- Try to minimize opening the oven to peek at your food, as this lets heat escape.

PANTRY PREP FOR A GRID-DOWN

Nonperishable foods boast extended shelf lives and do not require refrigeration to stay safe to eat. This translates to convenience, with quick meals or snacks at your fingertips and peace of mind, knowing you are prepared for a grid-down. Look at this list of nonperishable food items for inspiration to stock up your pantry:

Category	Options
Canned goods	• canned fish such as sardines or tuna
	• canned meat such as chicken or beef
	• canned fruits such as peaches, pears, or pineapples
	• canned beans such as kidney and black beans
	• canned vegetables such as green beans or corn
Dried foods	• grains and starches such as pasta, rice, conscious, oats, or quinoa
	• dried beans and legumes such as pinto beans, lentils, or split peas
	• dried vegetables such as mushrooms, corn, onions, or garlic
	• dried meat such as jerky or dried sausage

Dehydrated or freeze-dried foods	• dehydrated fruits and vegetables such as apple slices, banana chips, mixed vegetables, or even mushrooms
	• dehydrated meals such as shepherd's pie, backpacking meals, or breakfast scrambles
	• freeze-dried berries, fruits like strawberries or mangos, and even apples
	• freeze-dried vegetables like peas, broccoli, or corn
Grains and cereals	• grains such as white rice, brown rice, rolled oats, barley, and farro
	• hot cereals such as cream of wheat or grits
	• cold cereals such as granola or granola bars
Nuts and nut butter	• Nuts such as almonds, peanuts, cashews, walnuts, or simply mixed nuts.
	• Nut butters such as peanut butter, almond butter, or cashew butter.
	• *Quick tip:* Opt for dry-roasted or unsalted butter whenever possible. Salted nuts can add unwanted sodium to your diet, and pre-flavored nuts often contain added sugars.
Natural sweeteners	Honey, maple syrup, dates, or coconut sugar

Milk	• shelf-stable milk
	• nondairy alternatives such as coconut milk or almond milk
Ready-to-eat meals	Freeze-dried camping meals, such as those rehydrated with hot water

Stocking the pantry with a well-thought-out food supply is the first thing to do. But how much is enough?

We recommend having *at least one week's worth* of nonperishable food for each person in your household. This provides a buffer while you wait for the power to be restored or for stores to reopen. It also gives you time to plan and cook meals without the pressure of daily grocery shopping.

Here are some factors to consider when calculating your needs:

- The number of people in the house.

- Do any household members have allergies or intolerances or follow specific diets? Stock items that cater to everyone's needs.

- Consider your typical calorie intake and adjust portions accordingly.

- Include some shelf-stable snacks, cookies, or treats for a morale boost.

MUST-HAVE MANUAL KITCHEN TOOLS FOR POWER OUTAGES

Tool	Use	Benefit
Manual can opener	Opens canned goods	Access to shelf-stable protein, vegetables, fruits, and precooked meals
Hand grinder	Grinds coffee beans, spices, and grains	Freshly ground coffee, customized spice blends, and the possibility of grinding grains for flour
Mortar and pestle	Grind spices and herbs and create pastes–marinades	Freshly ground spices for maximum flavor; creation of homemade spice rubs and pastes
Hand crank blender	Blends purees and chops ingredients	Ability to make soups, sauces, salsas, dips, and pestos without electricity
Box grater	Grates cheese, vegetables, and fruits	Freshly grated cheese for pasta dishes, toppings, or salads. Zesting citrus fruits for baking or drinks.

PRESERVING FOOD IN AN OUTAGE

Keeping food fresh can be challenging without a fridge. Here are some clever ways to extend the shelf life of your limited supplies and prevent them from spoiling through preservation.

CANNING

Canning is "a time-tested method that uses heat to destroy spoilage enzymes and bacteria in food. It then creates a vacuum seal in jars to prevent new bacteria from entering." This allows for safe storage of fruits, vegetables, and even meats for extended periods.

Boiling Water Bath Canning
- **Perfect for:** High-acid foods such as fruits, jams, jellies, and pickles—vinegar-based)

- **Why it works:** High-acid foods naturally inhibit bacterial growth. It makes the boiling water bath's heat sufficient for safe preservation. It heats the jars to a temperature that destroys harmful microorganisms. The seal prevents air from spoiling the food.

The Process
Step 1: Gather Your Supplies

- **Canning jars** (mason jars or other canning-approved jars)

- **Lids and bands**

- **Large pot or canner** (big enough to fully submerge your jars with at least 1 inch of water above the jars)

- **Jar lifter or tongs** (to safely handle hot jars)

- **Funnel** (for filling jars without spilling)

- **Bubble remover tool or plastic spatula** (to remove air bubbles from the jars)

- **Clean towel or cloth** (for wiping jar rims)

- **Timer** (to keep track of the processing time)

Step 2: Prepare your Jars and Lids

Wash the Jars: Carefully clean your jars and lids with hot water and soap and ensure they are free of cracks

Sterilize Jars:

- Place the jars in a pot of water and bring it to a boil for 10 minutes.

- Keep them warm in hot water until you're ready to use them. This prevents jar breakage from thermal shock.

Prepare Lids: If you're using new, metal canning lids (which is recommended for safety), you don't need to sterilize them. However, you should **soften** the sealing compound by simmering the lids in hot water (not boiling) for about 5 minutes before use. Don't boil them, as it can damage the rubber seal.

Step 3: Prepare Your Food

1. **Fill Jars**:

   o Use a **funnel** to carefully pour the prepared food into the warm jars, leaving the appropriate **headspace** (usually 1/4 to 1/2 inch) between the food and the jar rim. This allows for expansion and proper sealing.

   o **Remove air bubbles**: Gently tap the jar on the counter or use a plastic spatula to remove air bubbles by running it around the inside edges of the jar.

   o Wipe the jar rims with a clean, damp towel to remove any food residue that could interfere with the sealing process.

2. **Apply Lids and Bands**:

   ○　Place the **lid** on top of the jar.

   ○　Screw the **band** on until it's just fingertip-tight. Don't over-tighten, as air needs to escape during the canning process.

Step 4: Boiling Water Bath Process

- **Fill the Canner with Water**: Fill a large pot with enough water to fully cover the jars by at least 1 inch. Bring the water to a **boil**.

- **Submerge the Jars**: Ensure the jars are submerged by at least 1 inch of water above the top. Use a **jar lifter** to carefully place the jars into the pots. Keep the jars from touching each other during the process (use a **canning rack** if you have one).

- **Boil for the Recommended Time**: Keep the water at a gentle boil between five to 45 minutes depending on the food you are canning, altitude or recipe you are using.

- **Maintain Water Levels**: If needed, add boiling water to the pot to keep the jars covered during the processing time.

Use a jar lifter to remove the jars from the boiling water. After processing, let the jars cool undisturbed for 12–24 hours.

Label with date and content and store in cool dry and dark place. Porperly sealed jars can last for up to a year.

Pressure Canning
- **Perfect for:** Low-acid foods such as vegetables, meats, and fish.

- **Why it works:** Low-acid foods require higher temperatures to destroy harmful bacteria. Pressure canners create a pressurized environment that reaches temperatures exceeding boiling water, which results in safe preservation.

The Process
- Follow your pressure canner's instructions for venting and adding water.

- Place filled jars with low-acid food on a rack in the pressure canner.

- Seal the canner and follow the manufacturer's instructions for reaching the recommended pressure—usually 10–15 lbs/sq in.

- Process the jars for the recommended time according to your recipe—can vary depending on the food.

- After processing, let the pressure canner cool down naturally and depressurize before opening.

- Let the jars cool undisturbed for 12–24 hours.

Tips for Canning
- Always follow a tested and reliable canning recipe for your chosen food.

- Both methods require checking for sealed lids after cooling. An unsealed jar indicates unsafe preservation, and the food should be refrigerated or reprocessed.

DEHYDRATING
Dehydration is "an ancient food preservation technique that removes moisture from food and slows down spoilage. It can be used with fruits, vegetables, herbs, and even meats."

How to Use a Dehydrator?

1. Start by preparing your food. Wash and thoroughly dry your fruits, vegetables, or herbs. Slice or chop your ingredients.

2. Arrange the pieces in a single layer on the dehydrator trays and make sure there is enough space between them for proper air circulation.

3. Set the right temperature and time by consulting your dehydrator's manual for recommended settings.

4. Let your dehydrator do the rest. It can take several hours, so you will have to be patient.

5. Once your food is dehydrated, store it in airtight containers in a cool, dark, and dry place.

FERMENTATION

Fermentation is a simple and reliable way to preserve food at home. It uses microorganisms such as bacteria and yeast to break down sugars and starches in a food to create beneficial by-products like lactic acid or alcohol. Fermentation also inhibits the growth of harmful bacteria. This process extends shelf life and adds unique flavors and textures.

How to Ferment Vegetables?

1. Find a cool, dark place. Aim for 60–65°F (16–18°C) and avoid areas near heat sources.

2. Use high-quality jars, such as clip-top jars with replaceable rubber seals.

3. Prepare a two-to-five-percent salt brine—by weight—for long-term storage.

4. Allow the water to cool to room temperature before adding it to the vegetables.

5. Cut vegetables into pieces and pack them tightly into jars. You can add garlic, dill, bay leaves or pepper corn. Cover with brine, and ensure it fully covers the vegetables.

6. Seal the jar with a **loose-fitting lid** or a fermentation lid that allows gases to escape. If you use a regular lid, you may need to loosen it up occasionally to allow gases to escape.

7. Store in a cool dark place.

Tips for Fermentation
- You can use raw honey and vinegar as a substitute for salt brine.

- Fruits can be fermented into cider or wine as well.

- Cold storage—below 50°F—allows you to use less salt in the brine.

PICKLING

Pickling "uses an acidic brine to inhibit the growth of bacteria. This process not only extends the shelf life of your produce but also adds a tangy and flavorful twist to the food."

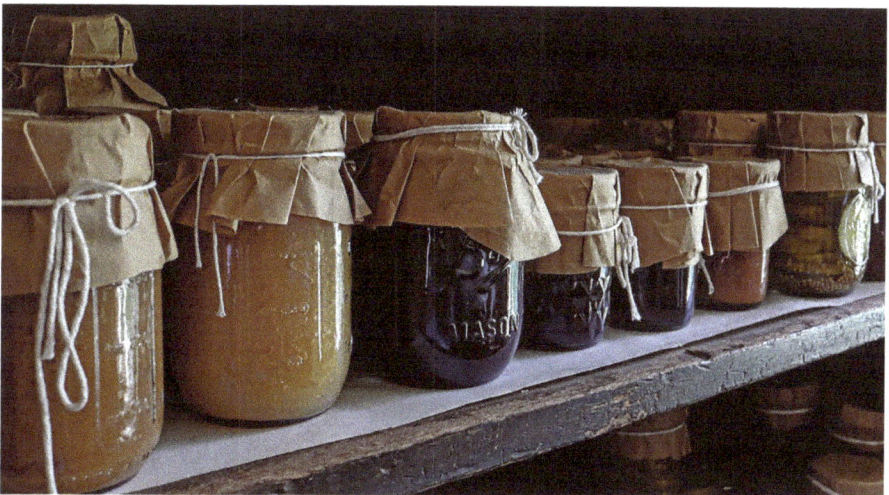

How to Pickle?

1. Wash and slice or chop your vegetables into desired shapes.

2. Combine water, vinegar, salt, and your chosen spices in a pot and bring to a boil. Let the brine cool slightly.

3. Place your prepared vegetables in a clear, sterilized jar. Fill the jar with cooled brine.

4. Wipe the rim of the jar clean and secure a lid tightly. Make sure to leave some headspace in the jar.

5. The pickling process will take anywhere from a few hours to several weeks, depending on the desired results. You can store your pickled vegetables at room temperature for a few days or weeks to allow the flavors to develop.

STORING FOOD THE RIGHT WAY

With your pantry stocked with carefully preserved vegetables, fruits, and other goodies, you might think your work is done. But there is one final step. Now that you have stocked the shelves, creating the right storage environment is needed. Here is how to do it:

- Store your food in a cool, dark place like a pantry, basement, or cabinet away from direct sunlight. Consistent temperatures work well, so avoid areas with fluctuating heat, such as near ovens or stoves.

- Place recent items behind older ones to make sure that you are using the older items first. This will help prevent expiration or spoilage.

- Moisture and pests are enemies of long-lasting food. Transfer opened packages or bags of food into airtight containers.

- Clear labeling will keep your pantry organized and prevent guesswork. Use labels with the contents and the date you acquired them.

- *Bonus:* Regularly assess your stockpile. Rotate your stock and replace items as needed.

START YOUR OWN GARDEN

Love fresh herbs and veggies and cannot imagine surviving without them in a grid-down? Your garden needs to be resilient and self-sufficient. Here are some quick tips to get you started:

- Pick a spot that gets sunshine for at least six to eight hours daily with good drainage. Raised beds can help if needed.

- Select an area close to a water source or rainwater catchment

- Start with easy-to-grow veggies and herbs like tomatoes, peppers, basil, or lettuce. They're less fussy and offer a quicker harvest.

- Improve the quality of the soil by composting and mulching

- If space allows, dwarf fruit trees are a great option for smaller areas. Plant, water deeply, and stake the tree for support.

- Choose crops that are hardy and do not require much care, that can be stored without refrigeration such as garlic, or squash

- Stock up on heirloom seeds

- Research specific needs for your chosen plants based on your climate—especially chilling hours. Your local gardening store or extension office can offer valuable advice.

TO SUM UP

Let's put your skills to the test and discover the possibilities of cooking in a grid-down. Using the methods suggested in this chapter, take a three-day challenge to cook without electricity. Can you cook rice over a campfire? Find out.

URBAN WATER SOURCING AND PURIFICATION

Water is essential for survival, even more so than food. For your family's well-being during a grid-down, it is important to have a reliable water supply. This chapter involves strategies to store enough water for immediate needs and develop alternative sources for long-term sustainability.

LEARNING OBJECTIVES

After reading this chapter, you will be able to:

- Develop strategies to find water during a power outage

- Learn how to properly store water for emergency use

- Understand methods to purify water if a safe source is unavailable

- Explore techniques on how to conserve or reuse water for hygiene, dishwashing, and other essentials

A STEP-BY-STEP GUIDE TO WATER PREPAREDNESS IN A GRID-DOWN

Unlike what you might see on the heavily scripted *reality shows* on TV, pulling gallons of water from thin air is not easy. Therefore, follow the steps outlined below to make sure you have enough water.

PLANNING

If you live in a house and can store water for a long time, it is wise to prepare and think how you are going to store water. Portable water containers can easily be taken with you in case of an evacuation. To avoid the growth of bacteria, refill them every six months. If you have the luxury of purchasing water barrel or tanks, they allow for larger amount of water.

STEP 01: ASSESSING WATER NEEDS

Before you grab a bucket and head for the nearest puddle, let's figure out how much water your household needs.

Count Heads

The first step in assessing your water needs is counting total water users. Do not forget to include your pets and, most importantly, yourself.

Calculate Daily Water Needs

Your daily water needs can be categorized into two main areas:

- **Essentials:** Aim for at least 1 gal of water per person per day for drinking, cooking, and preparing beverages.

- **Hygiene:** Allocate an additional 1–2 gal per person daily for tasks like handwashing, dishwashing, and personal hygiene.

Let's use an example: a family of four, including two adults and two children. Here's a rough estimate of their daily water needs:

1. **Essentials:** 4 people x 1 gal/person = 4 gal/day

2. **Hygiene:** 4 people x 1.5 gal/person (average) = 6 gal/day

3. **Total daily requirement:** 4 gal/day (essentials) + 6 gal/day (hygiene) = 10 gal/day

Keep Building Your Stockpile
Now, you know how much water your household needs daily. But how much should you actually store? Here's where planning comes in.

- Aim for a minimum of a two-week supply initially. This buffer gives you time to find alternative water sources if needed.

- Keep expanding your water storage as you become more prepared. Maybe you can dedicate additional space in your basement or garage for extra water containers.

STEP 02: STORING WATER
You know how much water each individual in your household needs, but now, how do you store it? Let's explore some of the best ways. Here are two main options:

Bottled Water
Commercially bottled water offers a readily available and easy-to-store option. Look for brands with a long shelf life and purchase them in bulk during sales.

Plastic water bottles, while convenient, are slightly permeable. This means tiny amounts of surrounding substances can seep through the plastic over time. To be sure that your water stays fresh and safe to drink, store bottled water away from household cleaning supplies and chemicals in a cool and dark place. These chemicals can potentially leach into the plastic and contaminate your water supply (Ajmera, 2020).

Food-Grade Containers
For a more cost-effective and long-term solution, invest in reusable food-grade containers. These come in various sizes and materials, like BPA-free plastic, glass, or even stainless steel.

Before filling your containers, wash them thoroughly with warm, soapy water or sanitize them with a bleach solution—1/4 teaspoon bleach per 1 qt of water; rinse thoroughly (Bodnar, 2021). This will help the water stay fresh and avoid any contamination.

Info-Bite
BPA stands for Bisphenol-A, a chemical sometimes used in the manufacturing of certain plastics. Concerns have been raised about the potential health effects of BPA, particularly at high exposure levels. While the science on BPA's health risks is debated, you can avoid it altogether (Bauer, 2023).

Water Storage Tips
- Regardless of your chosen storage method, keep your water containers in a cool, dark place. Sunlight can promote algae growth and degrade plastic containers, while extreme temperatures can affect the taste.

- Avoid storing water near heat sources like ovens or in areas prone to freezing temperatures. Both can damage the containers.

- Water has a shelf life (Ajmera, 2020). Therefore, it is advised to rotate your water supplies every six months. Drink the older water first and replace it with fresh water.

STEP 03: COLLECTING WATER

While bottled water and containers offer a great starting point, there are ways to become more self-sufficient when it comes to water security. Here are some additional methods to collect water for usage:

Rainwater Harvesting

Rainwater harvesting is a fantastic way to collect free, clean water. Here is how this can be done:

1. Identify the surface that will collect the rainwater. This is your catchment area. It could be your rooftop, a paved courtyard, or even unpaved ground. Choose an area that receives good rainfall and is easy to clean. A clean catchment area results in cleaner rainwater for storage.

2. Next, think about the physical setup. This includes the location of your storage tank and the pipelines that will transport the collected water. There are different options, but two popular ones include a spread-out tank option—one large tank positioned strategically near your catchment area—and a cluster tank option—multiple smaller tanks, potentially positioned at different locations.

3. The collected rainwater needs a safe place to store. This is where a storage tank comes in. The size and design of your tank will depend on your water needs, the average rainfall in your area, and the size of your catchment area.

4. When setting up your rainwater storage tank, know you can use a double whammy for cleanliness. A mesh filter stops debris, while a *first flush* diverter excludes the initial dirty rainwater that washes off your catchment area. For even cleaner water, consider installing a filtration system before the storage tank.

5. Now, connect the different components of your rainwater harvesting system. Check with local authorities if any permits are needed for laying pipes on your property. If your pipes will be underground, you will need to dig trenches to accommodate them. Once pipes are laid, use connectors to link them together.

6. To install a tank, create a stable stand by considering its weight when empty. Secure the tank on the stand and make sure it won't topple over when empty.

7. Set up an overflow system to prevent tank overfilling. This may involve additional drainage if the tanks are in a sump.

8. Connect the PVC collector pipes to the storage tank(s).

9. Finally, install a tank gauge to monitor your water level and usage.

Natural Water Sources
Before a crisis hits, identify potential water sources within a 5-mi radius of your house. You must know that carrying heavy water containers long distances is a challenge. Here is what to consider:

- Ideally, find water sources upstream from farms or industrial areas to avoid contamination from runoff.

- Explore all possibilities, including lakes, ponds, rivers, streams, and springs.

- Consider ways to collect and transport water. You can invest in jerricans or stackable water jugs with handles. These hold large volumes and make transport easier.

- Assess factors like distance, terrain, and potential hazards when identifying natural water sources. Keep more than one option in mind.

- *Must-know:* Regulations regarding water use from natural sources may apply. Check with your local authorities to understand any restrictions on collecting water from lakes, rivers, streams, or springs in your area.

Emergency Water Sources
In an absolute pinch, you can potentially collect small amounts of water from unexpected household items, such as:

Hot Water Heater
A hot water heater can serve as an emergency source of water. Here's how:

- Find your heater—basement or garage for houses, closets for apartments—and determine whether it's electric or natural gas—look for vent, pilot light, and gas line.

- Shut off the heater's power source and the water supply valve—usually on top of the heater.

- Open the pressure relief valve on the heater tank or turn on hot water faucets elsewhere in the house to release air from the tank.

- Place a container under the drain valve at the bottom of the heater. Wear gloves and safety glasses, and carefully open the valve—it might be hot!—to drain the water. Repeat until empty.

Melted Ice Cubes
You can also use melted ice cubes, but only if they are made from clean, uncontaminated water. Purify the melted water before drinking.

Commercially Bottled Beverages
Consider juice, sodas, or other drinks that you might have, but be mindful that caffeinated and alcoholic drinks can dehydrate you, so consume them sparingly.

Canned Fruits and Vegetables

Look for options packed in water. In an emergency, liquids from canned foods can be consumed if necessary. However, never consume beverages or canned food from containers that have been flooded.

How to Test Water for Contamination?

Testing water quality can help you determine if it is safe to drink or not. Water test strips, like those found in the Health Metric Test Kit, are a common choice because they are affordable and easy to use, even without electricity.

Although the specific instructions might vary slightly by brand, here are some steps on how to do it:

1. Gather your supplies. You will need a clean container for your water sample, the test strip, and the kit's color chart.

2. Fill the container with the water you want to test.

3. Dip the test strip into the water sample, following the kit's instructions on how long to hold it submerged. Swirl the container gently to mix the water.

4. Let the test strip sit for the recommended time. Then, compare the color changes on the strip to the color chart provided in the kit.

5. The color chart will explain what the different colors on the test strip indicate about potential contamination levels.

Tips

- Only open test strips when you are ready to use them. Exposure to air can affect accuracy.

- Wash your hands thoroughly before handling the test strip.

- Use cold water for the sample. If you only have access to hot water, let it cool down first.

- If the results show contamination, you can use the purification methods outlined in the next step, test again, and consume the water.

STEP 04: PURIFYING WATER

Even seemingly clean water sources like ponds or streams can have harmful viruses that are invisible and undetectable. While most purifiers promise to eliminate up to 99.9% of these viruses and bacteria, that is the best you will get in an emergency. Therefore, do not take a chance with your health, and always purify water before using it from questionable sources.

Filtration

The filtration process removes impurities like rust, parasites, sediment, and bacteria from the liquid. You can opt for the following:

Type	Use	Example
Portable water filter	• Perfect for individual use. Compact and lightweight for portability. • Works by forcing water through a filter, trapping contaminants like bacteria and parasites. • Ideal to purify water on the go.	• LifeStraw • Sawyer Mini

Gravity-fed filtration system	• Designed for larger groups or steady water supply needs	• SimPure Gravity Water Filter
	• Uses gravity to slowly filter water through stages like sediment and carbon filters	• PureWell 304 Stainless Steel Gravity-Fed Water Filter
	• Good choice for areas with a longer stay	

Boiling
The *Centers for Disease Control and Prevention* suggests bringing your water to a full rolling boil for 1 minute or 3 minutes if you are above 6,500 ft. Before using it, let it cool completely (*Boil Water Advisory*, 2023).

If you can, boil even filtered water to add extra protection.

Do not forget that pets can also catch waterborne illnesses. Give them bottled water or cooled, boiled water to drink.

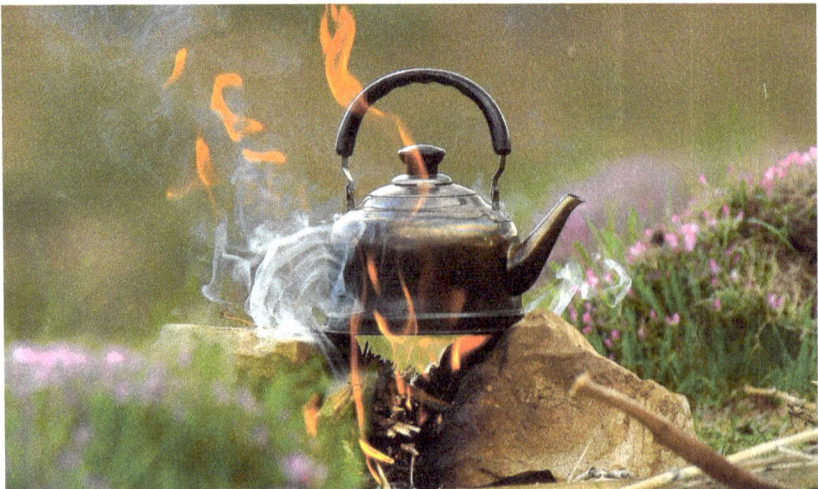

Info-Bite

A *boil water advisory* is "a safety measure issued by local authorities when there is a chance that your tap water might be contaminated." This usually happens during power outages because pumps that treat and distribute water may not function properly. To be clear, the advisory recommends boiling your tap water to kill any harmful bacteria.

Chemical Purification

Chemical purification can be done using the following methods:

- Water purification tablets that come in chlorine and iodine versions. Chlorine tablets are user-friendly and effective but may leave a slight chlorine taste. Iodine tablets have a longer shelf life, but people with shellfish allergies should avoid them as they can trigger an allergic reaction.

- Bleach is another powerful disinfectant for water purification, though its effectiveness wanes after only 6 months. Careful storage and precise measurement (8–16 drops/gal) are important. Liquid iodine offers a longer shelf life compared to bleach but requires a higher dosage per gallon (20–40 drops). The quantity depends on various factors such as the impurity of water and the strength of bleach, therefore, before using it, read the manufacturer's instructions very carefully.

UV Purification

Might sound a bit fancy, but UV light devices like SteriPEN offer a convenient option. They use ultraviolet light to zap bacteria and parasites from your water and make it safe to drink. However, for best results, the water needs to be clear. Cloudiness or sediment can block the UV light and prevent it from reaching all the contaminants.

STEP 05: STORING WATER FOR HYGIENE

It is essential to maintain good hygiene to prevent illness even in a grid-down. Do not risk mixing non-potable—hygiene—and drinking water. Designate separate, clearly labeled containers for hygiene purposes. Since you will need more for washing than drinking, consider large, food-grade containers for bulk storage. For daily use, fill smaller jugs or collapsible containers. Don't forget to label them "Hygiene Water" to avoid confusion.

STEP 06: SAVING WATER THROUGH ALTERNATIVES

We've outlined some tips for you to save water whenever and wherever possible.

For Hygiene

- Wash hands with soap and clean water whenever possible. But, to save water, prioritize using a small amount of water and soap for a quick wash, then finish with a hand sanitizer.

- Skip the shower. Opt for a sponge bath instead. Use a washcloth and a small amount of soapy water to clean your body.

- Dry shampoo can be your friend. It helps freshen hair in between washes.

- Use a cup of water to rinse your mouth after brushing instead of letting the tap run.

- Try shaving with a damp washcloth instead of running water.

For Toilets

- If you have land, consider building an outhouse for long-term waste disposal. Even a simple pit latrine—a hole with a seat—can work, but remember to dig it away from water sources and fill it when full.

- For indoor use, line a 5-gal bucket with a heavy-duty trash bag. Keep the lid on when not in use to minimize odor, and change the bag daily or when it gets full.

- In case of limited water but a functioning toilet, consider manual flushing with a gallon of water.

For Dishwashing
- Use the two-bucket method. Fill one bucket with soapy water for washing dishes. Fill another bucket with clean water treated with a few drops of bleach for rinsing.

- Consider using individually wrapped plastic cutlery—forks, spoons, and knives—to avoid washing dishes. Opt for single-use or daily-use sets.

For Trash
- Invest in heavy-duty garbage bags to handle waste effectively.

- Regularly remove trash from your home to prevent unpleasant odors, maggot infestations, and other hazards.

- Keep trash containers away from your house and water sources to avoid contamination.

- Burning is also an option if done with caution. Only burn paper and natural materials. Avoid burning plastics or chemical containers due to harmful fumes.

- If other options are unavailable, bury trash at least 100 ft away from water sources. Dig a deep hole, at least 18 in., to prevent animals from digging it up.

Recycle Your Water

Do not let the used water go down the drain. Here is how you can reuse it:

- Use pasta or rice water for soups, sauces, or watering nonedible plants.

- Dishwater from the first rinse—before soap—can be used for cleaning any spills in the house or mopping floors.

- After rinsing fruits and vegetables, collect the water to wash your hands, only if you can sanitize them later.

STEP 07: CREATING A BACKUP PLAN

For reliable access to clean water during an emergency, aim for redundancy in both storage and purification methods.

Store water in various locations throughout your home. Use the space under sinks and bathtubs or even fill spare containers. Moreover, consider off-site storage at a friend's place or garage if feasible. This helps create a buffer if your primary location becomes inaccessible in case of a natural disaster.

When it comes to purification, do not rely on a single method. Keep extra filters and stock of tablets to have a backup if your primary method fails or you run out of supplies.

STEP 08: MAINTENANCE AND ROTATION

As a final layer of protection, do not let your water sit and forget. Regularly inspect all your stored water containers for leaks, cracks, or signs of contamination. Check your rainwater collection systems—if applicable—to see if they are working properly and free of debris.

Stored water is not meant to last forever. As a general rule, replace your stored water every six months. This helps maintain freshness and taste. Clearly label your water containers with the date they were filled. This will help you easily identify which ones need to be replaced first.

TO SUM UP

Maintaining a clean and healthy environment can be a challenge without water. Follow the eight steps outlined above to handle a power outage with minimal disruption to your family's access to water.

5

EVACUATION ESSENTIALS—YOUR GO-BAG CHECKLIST

To evacuate or to stay put when an emergency strikes? What do you take along with you? How do you develop an evacuation plan for the family? This chapter has all the answers to your evacuation-related questions.

LEARNING OBJECTIVES

This chapter explores:

- Steps to take during an emergency evacuation

- How to develop an evacuation plan for your household

- Items to include in your evacuation go-bag

- Tips for maintaining and updating your evacuation bag for maximum preparedness

WHEN TO EVACUATE?

Disasters come in many forms, and knowing when to evacuate is important for your safety. Here are some key triggers:

OFFICIAL ALERTS

Listen closely to broadcasts on radio or mobile news apps. Text alerts from the emergency alert system might also instruct you to evacuate. These official warnings from police, fire departments, or local authorities take priority.

EVACUATION ORDERS

Instructions might be to evacuate entirely or to shelter-in-place by sealing off your home. Always follow the specific guidance provided by officials.

SEVERITY OF THE THREAT

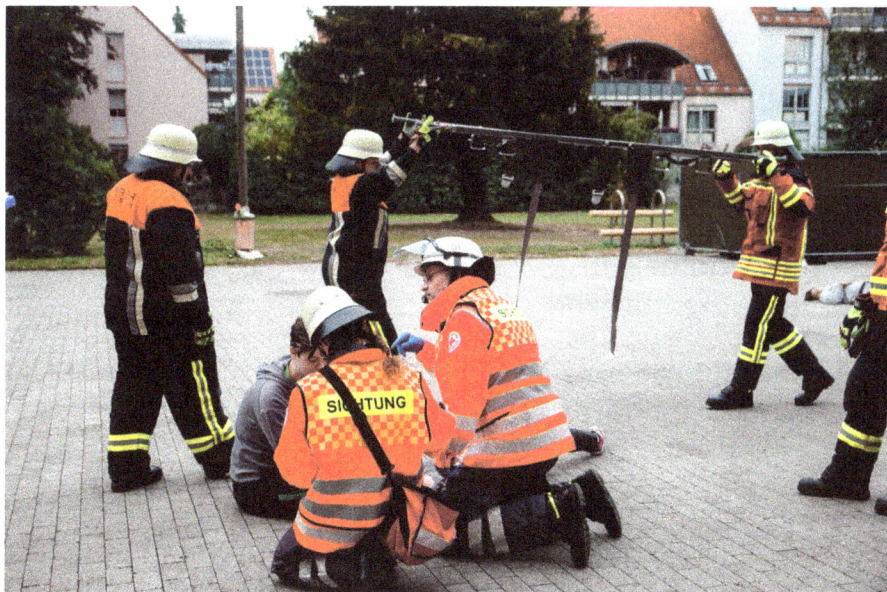

Evacuation decisions depend on the danger. Floods, hurricanes, tornadoes, and fires typically require evacuation. Chemical spills, gas leakage, and civil unrest might also necessitate leaving the area.

HOW TO DEVELOP AN EVACUATION PLAN?

In order to quickly and safely evacuate from your house in case of an emergency, you must have an evacuation plan ready. Here is a step-by-step process to design one:

STEP 01: ASSESS THE RISKS

- Identify the emergencies most likely to threaten your location. This could include floods, fires, tornadoes, or hurricanes.

- Consider your home's specific vulnerabilities. Does it lie in a floodplain? Is it prone to wildfires? Understanding the risks will help you prepare the most effective evacuation plan.

STEP 02: DESIGNATE ESCAPE ROUTES

- Identify at least two escape routes from each room in your home. This will ensure you have options if one exit becomes blocked during an emergency.

- Include windows as potential escape routes, especially on upper floors. Check to see if the windows are easy to open and accessible in case of fire or other emergencies.

- Light up your escape routes for a grid-down. Consider installing motion-activated LED lights for hands-free illumination. Additionally, glow-in-the-dark strips or stickers placed strategically on walls, door handles, and along corridors can provide extra visibility in low-light conditions.

- Secure bookshelves, cabinets, and other large furniture pieces to the wall studs using heavy-duty brackets and screws. This prevents them from toppling over and causing injuries or blocking escape routes.

- Keep hallways and stairwells clear of clutter, furniture, and debris.

- Regularly check for any damage or malfunction in doors, locks, or windows. Fix any issues promptly. Moreover, consider installing sturdy door reinforcement kits for additional security.

- Walk through each escape route with your family to ensure they are clear and easy to reach, even in darkness.

STEP 03: CHOOSE A MEETING PLACE

- Select a safe meeting place outside your house, a good distance away from potential hazards like downed power lines or flooding.

- Consider your neighborhood layout and choose a location easily accessible for everyone in the family.

Review the following when deciding on a meeting point:

- Is the area located away from potential dangers?

- Is the area well-lit, especially at night?

- Can emergency responders reach the area easily?

- Does the area have good cell phone reception?

- Is the assembly point easy for everyone in your family to locate?

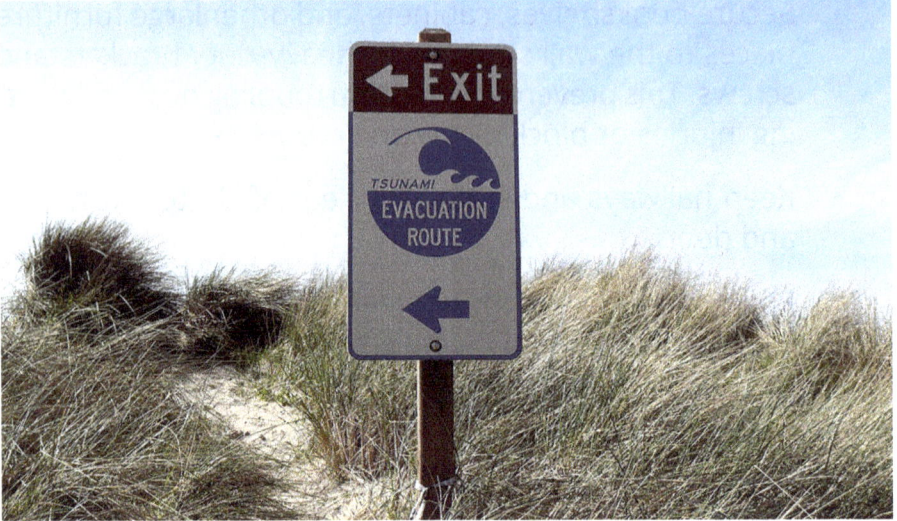

STEP 04: PACK AN EVACUATION BAG

Prepare a well-stocked evacuation bag for each member of your family. We'll discuss what to include in the bag later in this chapter. Consider keeping them by the designated exit for quick grab-and-go readiness.

STEP 05: PRACTICE MAKES PERFECT

Conduct a regular evacuation drill with your family. Practice using the decided escape routes and meeting at your chosen assembly point. You can do these drills both during the day and at night to ensure that everyone is comfortable in various lighting conditions. Regular practice familiarizes everyone with the plan and reduces confusion during a real emergency.

STEP 06: STAY INFORMED AND UPDATE YOUR EVACUATION PLAN

Monitor weather reports and emergency alerts closely, especially during times of heightened risk. In order to stay informed about evacuation orders issued by local authorities, make sure you do the following:

- Check with your local emergency management office to find out if your area has a Reverse Dial system and how to register. These systems can send prerecorded phone calls, emails, and text messages with instructions like evacuation orders, shelter locations, and safety updates.

- Include all your phone numbers (landline and cell), email address, and any other relevant contact details.

- Be aware of the limitations because the Reverse Dial is not available in all countries. Many areas use social media, public sirens, or community radio broadcasts to disseminate emergency information. Familiarize yourself with these additional channels.

ORGANIZING AND PREPARING YOUR EVACUATION GO-BAG

A *go bag*, also known as a *bug-out* bag or *emergency kit*, is "a portable collection of essential supplies you grab in a hurry during an emergency evacuation. It's designed to sustain you for a set period, typically three days until help arrives or you can return home."

EVACUATION GO-BAG CHECKLIST

- ❑ Water bottle and water filter

- ❑ Nonperishable food items such as ready-to-eat meals or freeze-dried items with a long shelf life

- ❑ Air filtration mask

- ❑ Change of clothes

- ❑ Cold weather gloves and a light-weight blanket

- ❑ Flashlight and headlights with extra batteries

- ❑ First aid kit

- ❑ Communication devices such as a two-way radio or mobile phone with batteries

- ❑ Charger or power bank for mobile, and batteries for radio
- ❑ Personal hygiene items such as tissue paper, soap, and hand sanitizer
- ❑ Fire-starting tools or matches
- ❑ Whistle to signal
- ❑ Local area and state maps
- ❑ Compass
- ❑ Fishing and sewing kit
- ❑ Family's prescription medications
- ❑ A multitool that comes with a knife, piler, can opener, and more
- ❑ Copies of important documents in an airtight container, including passports, titles and contracts, IDs, proof of address, and phone numbers of loved ones for communication
- ❑ Emergency cash of at least $500
- ❑ Extra keys to your house

If applicable:

- ❑ Toddler supplies, including diapers and feeding bottles
- ❑ Pet supplies, such as leashes and pet food

VEHICLE EMERGENCY KIT CHECKLIST

It is suggested that you keep an emergency kit in your vehicle in case you are unable to return home during a disaster. It should include:

- ❑ Water bottles—at least 1 gal/person
- ❑ Nonperishable food

- ❑ Blanket

- ❑ Extra clothing and shoes

- ❑ First aid kit

- ❑ Seat belt cutter

- ❑ Candles in deep metal cans and matches

- ❑ Wind-up flashlight

- ❑ Road maps

- ❑ Whistle

- ❑ Copy of important documents

HOW TO PUT YOUR EVACUATION BAG TOGETHER?

Having a checklist is not enough. Follow these steps to organize and prepare a go-bag for evacuation:

- Select a sturdy, waterproof backpack with multiple compartments for easy organization.

- Consider a backpack with a built-in water reservoir for easy access to hydration.

- Place important items like water, food, a first aid kit, and communication tools in the closest compartments.

- Distribute weight evenly to make carrying the bag more manageable.

- Label compartments or use color-coded bags for quick identification of items.

- Pack delicate items in protective cases or wrap them in clothing to prevent damage.

TIPS FOR MAINTAINING AND UPDATING YOUR EVACUATION BAG

Preparing a go-bag is just the beginning. Therefore, it's essential to do the following:

- Replace food and water supplies nearing expiration and update clothing according to seasonal changes.

- Update copies of important documents, including identification, medical records, and emergency contacts.

- Consider changes in family size or specific needs—like medications or dietary restrictions—when updating supplies.

- Stay updated on local emergency protocols and adjust your bag contents accordingly.

TO SUM UP

With an evacuation plan and go-bag in place, you are now ready to face emergencies better. Print the checklists provided in this chapter and tick the items as you prepare your go bag. By taking action now, you and your family can stay safe during unsettling times.

6

TINY TOT PREPAREDNESS— ENSURING INFANT SAFETY IN CRISIS

Sleepless nights, endless feedings, and the constant demands of a tiny human can be overwhelming under normal circumstances, let alone a grid-down situation. This chapter offers practical advice and strategies to care for your baby during a power outage.

LEARNING OBJECTIVES

In this chapter:

- Learn practical solutions to replace essential supplies for your baby through available resources and alternative methods.

- Explore techniques to maintain your baby's hygiene without regular access to water.

- Gain knowledge to prepare an emergency kit tailored for an infant.

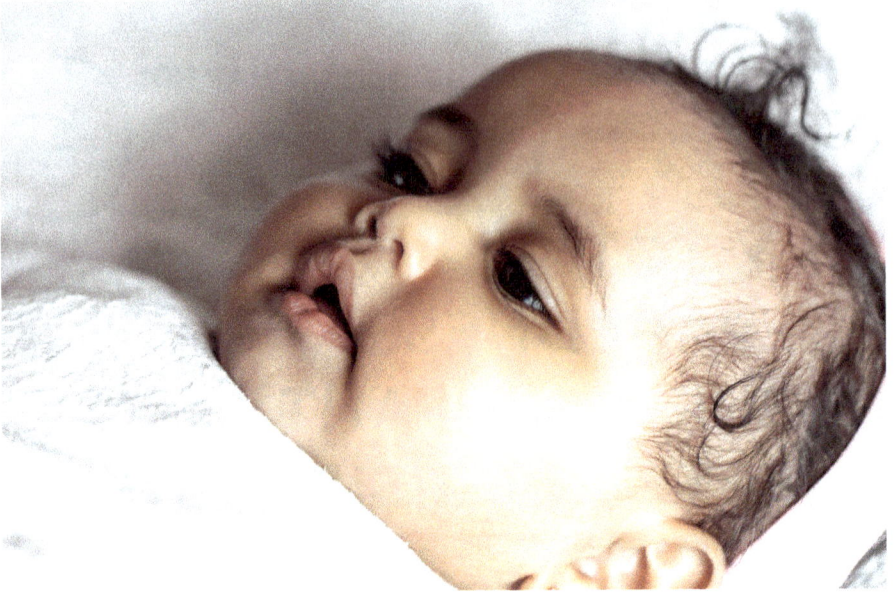

RUNNING OUT OF ESSENTIALS

In a grid-down scenario, running out of essential supplies, such as diapers, wipes, baby food, and medications, can become a challenge for your baby's health. Preparing for the situation involves understanding the potential problems and exploring suitable solutions. Let's take a look.

PROBLEM 01
You have run out of diapers.

SOLUTION
In emergencies, you can repurpose old cotton T-shirts, towels, or bed sheets into makeshift diapers. Make sure that the cloth is clean and soft to the touch. You can also use flannel receiving blankets as a base and secure them with safety pins or cloth diaper fasteners for a customized fit. If that is not an option, take advantage of elimination communication.

Elimination communication is based on observing your baby's cues to eliminate. Some common signs are:

- Squirming or fussing that could indicate discomfort and urge to eliminate

- Stiffening or pushing

- Older babies may squat when they need to go

- Some babies may try to hide when they are about to eliminate

- Grimacing or straining

- Focused or intense look on the face

PROBLEM 02
No more wipes in the stock.

SOLUTION
Similar to cloth diapers, you can use soft clothes or cut up old garments to make cloth wipes. To create homemade wipes:

1. Cut soft clothes into pieces of the desired size.

2. Soak the pieces in water and mild soap.

3. Add a few drops of essential oil.

4. Store them in a sealed container to keep them moist.

PROBLEM 03
Formula milk has been expired or damaged.

SOLUTION
In the event that formula milk is expired or damaged, searching for an alternative becomes important. Meanwhile, breastfeeding is the best possible nourishment for babies, especially

during emergencies, due to its immune-boosting character-istics. However, many women who use formula may not be producing breast milk. Following are some fill-in measures to ponder:

Milk Bank
Consider reaching out to your local milk bank, as some pro-vide breast milk without a prescription. Begin by introducing yourself and explaining your situation. Provide specific de-tails about your child, including age and any health concerns. Inquire about the process, availability, and any requirements to obtain the milk. Ask about safety and handling procedures to be sure the milk is suitable for your baby.

Re-Lactation
If you have recently stopped breastfeeding, *re-lactation* might be possible. Seek advice from a lactation consultant or health-care provider in advance to understand the steps and efforts required. Here are some tips for *re-lactation*:

- Boost your breast stimulation through pumping, hand expressing, or breastfeeding frequently.

- Ensure your baby latches on correctly to maximize milk transfer and stimulate production. Gentle breast mas-sage before and during feedings can help.

- Skin-to-skin contact can allow your baby to explore your breast and naturally encourage milk production.

- Use relaxation techniques to reduce your stress levels, which positively impacts your milk supply.

Community Support
Local support groups and community networks might have mothers willing to donate breast milk. However, when sourc-ing, ensure the milk is handled and stored safely.

Tip

Do not make your own formula. Homemade formula is not a safe alternative to commercial formula.

PROBLEM 04

The electrical breast pump is not working due to electricity shortage.

SOLUTION

Breast milk is the ideal nourishment for infants, especially during emergencies when the risk of disease is heightened due to contaminated water and unsanitary conditions. Breastfeeding provides vital antibodies that shield babies from common illnesses such as diarrhea and respiratory infections.

However, your electrical breast pump will fail to work in a grid-down. Here are two options to go for:

Use a Manual Pump

Follow the instructions provided with your specific pump. Sit or recline in a relaxed position. Make sure the nipple is centered in the breast shield for optimal suction. Gently compress the handle of the pump to mimic a baby's sucking rhythm. You may experience a let-down, which is when milk starts to flow more freely. Continue pumping until the milk flow slows or stops. Alternate between breasts to maximize milk output.

Use Hand Expression Technique

Start by washing your hands thoroughly with soap and water. Gently massage your breast to stimulate milk flow. Using your thumb and index fingers, form a "C" shape around your nipple. Apply gentle pressure toward your chest wall and release. Use a clean container to collect the expressed milk.

PROBLEM 05

Little to no medicines left.

SOLUTION

Running out of medications, especially for chronic conditions, can be life-threatening for your baby. To eliminate the risk, it is important to build a reserve of essential medications. Focus on those required for chronic conditions. Rotate the stock for freshness and consult a health care professional for guidance on safe storage.

It is good to know some natural remedies and alternative treatments for common ailments, such as the following:

Ear Infections
- Use hot and cold compresses alternatively to ease ear pain. A warm compress reduces inflammation, while a cold one numbs the area. Soak a clean cloth in warm or cold water, wring it out, and gently apply it to your child's ear. Switch between the two for effective pain relief.

- DIY garlic oil for ear infections: Crush two to three cloves of garlic and heat them gently in two tablespoons of olive oil until the garlic is fragrant. Allow the oil to cool, and then strain out the garlic pieces. Apply ear drops to the outer ear canal. Avoid inserting the dropper directly into the ear.

Skin Rash
- Apply a thin layer of coconut oil to the affected area. Coconut oil has natural antifungal and antibacterial properties, which can help soothe and heal diaper rash.

- If coconut oil is not available, use pure aloe vera gel directly onto the rash to reduce inflammation and promote healing.

Teething Relief
Dilute a small amount of clove oil with a carrier oil such as coconut oil and gently rub on the baby's gums. Clove oil has natural analgesic properties.

Tummy Aches
Ginger tea to the rescue! Grate a small piece of ginger and boil it in water. After it cools, give your baby a few sips to help with nausea and digestion.

PROBLEM 06
The baby monitor is not working without electricity.

SOLUTION
The safest option is to sleep in the same room as your baby. However, if that is not possible for you, consider:

- Storing portable battery packs that work well with battery-powered baby monitors

- Keeping visual check-in

- Paying close attention to sounds from your baby's room

PROBLEM 07
Limited ability to bathe the infant.

SOLUTION
Here is what you can do without having to use water:

Sponge Bath
Use a small amount of water and a clean sponge or washcloth to gently clean the baby. Focus on the face, neck, hands, diaper area, and any skin folds where dirt and bacteria can accumulate. Before giving a sponge bath, keep the baby in a warm area to prevent chills.

Dry Bath
Opt for a baby-safe dry shampoo and body powders to absorb oils and sweat. You can also use baby wipes for quick clean-ups. Choose wipes that are alcohol-free and designed for sensitive skin to avoid irritation.

Air Bath
Give your baby some time each day without a diaper. It will allow their skin to air out and breathe. This helps prevent rashes
and irritation caused by prolonged exposure to moisture.

PROBLEM 08
Struggle to dispose of diapers and used wipes.

SOLUTION
Double-bag the diapers by placing them into a thick, leak-proof
plastic bag. Encase the first bag into another larger bag. Tie
both bags tightly to prevent leaks and odors.

   If you have access to a suitable outdoor area, dig a deep
hole and bury the bagged diapers. Make the hole far from water sources to prevent contamination. Cover the hole with soil
to minimize odor and attractants.

PREPARING AN EMERGENCY EVACUATION KIT FOR YOUR BABY

Evacuating with a baby requires careful planning and preparation for their safety and comfort. Here is what to keep in your
infant emergency kit for scenarios such as a grid-down:

- ❑ Diapers and wipes

- ❑ Diaper rash cream

- ❑ Formula or breast milk

- ❑ Bottles and nipples, manual breast pumps

- ❑ Baby food and snacks

- ❑ Extra clothing and blankets

- ❑ Pacifiers and comfort items

- ❑ Baby first aid kit

- ❑ Car seat or carrier
- ❑ Contact information for pediatricians and hospitals
- ❑ Safety instructions for CPR and choking

BABY FIRST AID KIT

Babies bump, bruise, and get sick easily. A grid-down can make a bad situation worse; therefore, have these essentials in the first aid kit for added peace of mind and quick care of your child:

- ❑ Rectal thermometer for taking your infant's temperature

- ❑ Nasal aspirator to clear stuffy noses

- ❑ Saline drops or spray to loosen mucus for easier suctioning

- ❑ Infant acetaminophen for fever or pain—safe after 12 weeks (Garvey, 2023)

- ❑ Bandages in various sizes for minor wounds

- ❑ Antibiotic ointment for minor cuts

- ❑ Medicine dropper for administering medication

- ❑ Nail clippers

- ❑ Gas drops to relieve gas discomfort

- ❑ Petroleum jelly for diaper rash or dry skin

TO SUM UP

Babies are resilient, but their comfort and safety largely depend on their caregivers. Therefore, make sure you are calm throughout the situation. By following the guidelines outlined in the chapter and practicing emergency preparedness, you can confidently go through the challenges of caring for your baby. You have got this!

FURRY FRIENDS AND FAMILY—PET SURVIVAL TACTICS

This chapter will guide you through some *pawsome* tips to keep your furry, feathered, or scaly friend safe and comfortable during stressful situations. From training and preparation to seeking support, we'll cover it all!

LEARNING OBJECTIVES

By the end of this chapter, you will be able to:

- Learn ways to keep your pet calm during stressful situations

- Assemble a pet disaster preparedness kit

- Develop an emergency network for pet care

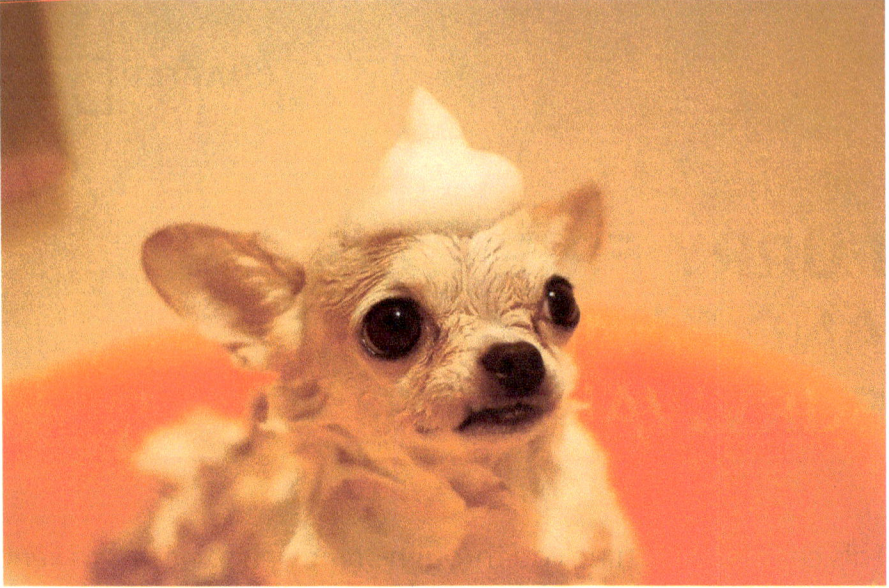

KEEPING YOUR PETS CALM DURING A GRID-DOWN

To keep your pets calm so they don't drive you up the wall with restlessness, do the following:

- Stock up on comfort foods like catnip for cats or other foods your pets are crazy about. You'll need to research safe alternatives.

- Get medication. A vet can give you drugs and supplements to desensitize or calm your pet in an emergency.

- Walk or exercise off the restlessness so that they're exhausted. This way, they'll lie down to rest and be still.

- Petting, grooming, playing, and talking with your pets can provide comfort and reduce their anxiety.

- Just like babies, pets sense your mood, so stay calm.

TRAINING YOUR PETS

If your pet can learn, teach them to respond to basic commands like how to sit, wait, follow, and even help you in a crisis. An obedient pet can stay out of your way well.

Do not forget to potty-train them and teach them skills like getting water for themself. The more low maintenance, the better!

For instance, as a dog owner, you can train your dog to respond to different commands.

Command	Importance in emergency
Sit	Keeps your dog in a safe place to prevent them from running off or into danger.
Come	Enables quick retrieval of the dog in an emergency situation.
Leave it	Prevents the dog from ingesting potentially harmful substances.
Wait	Helps control the dog in chaotic or unfamiliar environments.

Here are some techniques to train your pets:

• Use positive reinforcement. Reward your pet for following instructions. Use back scratches, toys, food, or praise.

• Understand that training takes time. Be patient and persistent, and do not get discouraged if your pet does not learn immediately. Celebrate small victories along the way.

• Make sure your pet can follow commands in different settings. Train them at home, in the park, and in other busy areas so that they can respond regardless of the location.

- Build it up in steps. Teach your cat to come to the tap to get a drink before showing them how to get their own.

BUILDING A SUPPORT NETWORK

A well-established support network provides peace of mind and ensures quick, coordinated action during a grid-down. To build a support network for your pet, follow these guidelines:

IDENTIFY LOCAL ORGANIZATIONS AND VOLUNTEERS

- Local organizations often have plans to provide temporary shelter, food, and medical care.

- Establish relationships with local vets who can offer emergency care and advice.

- Familiarize yourself with the local government's emergency plans for pets or reach out to the community volunteer groups for animal welfare well in advance.

USE PET CARE SERVICES

Consider boarding your pet in a secure facility if evacuation is needed. If you must evacuate and cannot take your pet, hire a reliable *petsitter*. In case of staying at your home, you can hire a mobile pet care service for your pets.

CONNECT WITH OTHER PET OWNERS

Sharing experiences and information with other pet owners can be beneficial. There are plenty of online forums and social media groups that you can join. Connect with pet owners in your area to exchange tips and support. Join local pet owner groups to build relationships and share resources. You can also get help from pet owners who have experienced similar emergencies in the past and ask for their advice.

MICROCHIPPING YOUR PET

Microchip your pets for their safe return if they become lost during an emergency. This tiny implant contains a unique identification number that can be scanned to locate your pet's information.

However, it's essential to verify that your pet's microchip information is accurate and up-to-date. Contact the microchip registration company to confirm your contact details and ensure your pet's record is complete. This proactive step can increase the chances of reuniting with your beloved companion in any emergency situation.

Regular check-ins with your pet's microchip registry are important, not just in a grid-down scenario but at all times.

CREATING A PET GO-BAG
FOR EMERGENCIES

When preparing your evacuation go-bag and stocking up supplies in your house for a grid-down, do not forget your pets. Here is a checklist to keep your pet safe and comfortable throughout an emergency:

- ❏ Nonperishable food items to last them for at least one week

- ❏ Clean drinking water

- ❏ Medicines for at least one week in advance

- ❏ Veterinary records, compiled as hard copies in a file, sorted by date

- ❏ Pet's first aid kit for minor injuries, including pain medications and tranquilizers, to last until you get them to a hospital

- ❏ Contact information for vets and pet-friendly shelters

❑ A list of contact numbers for fellow pet owners in your area who can offer support and share resources

❑ Extra leash and pet carrier or crate to keep them tied to you

❑ Grooming supplies for their hygiene

❑ Good-condition collar and ID tags with your details

❑ Extra tag for a secondary contact in case you are unavailable

❑ A recent photo of your pet to help track them

❑ A tracker with a long-term battery

❑ Comfort toys and food

SAFE TRAVELING WITH YOUR PET

If you need to evacuate with your pet, a carrier will be needed for sure. To reduce their stress during travel, familiarize them with their carrier beforehand.

• Place the carrier in a familiar area. Leave it open in a spot your pet frequents.

• Make it inviting by adding a soft blanket or bed to the carrier, and include treats inside.

• Feed your pet near the carrier to create positive connections.

• During travel, securely fasten carriers or crates to prevent movement during sudden stops.

• Avoid front seats, as back seats are safe for pets in case of accidents. Allow your pets to stretch and relieve themselves by adding regular breaks during the travel.

• Never leave your pets unattended in the car.

TO SUM UP

When things go south, your companions in crisis become a huge source of comfort. However, you also have to prepare supplies for your pet companions because they're your re-sponsibility. Once you're prepped for the comfort of everyone important to you, you're ready to face any grid-down crisis head-on!

CHAPTER 8

FIRST AID AND CPR

As you review these first aid and CPR skills, understand that different organizations have different standards and techniques that change over time. The skills provided below meet the Red Cross standards.

CPR

INTRODUCTION

Heart diseases, stroke, and cardiovascular diseases are still the number one cause of death in the US and increasing worldwide. Knowing what to do and taking prompt action when a loved one is in distress can make the difference between life and death.

LEARNING OBJECTIVES

After reading this chapter, you will be able to:

- Recognize the signs and symptoms of a heart attack in men and women

- Perform CPR on adults, children, and infants

SIGNS AND SYMPTOMS OF A HEART ATTACK

Below are the common signs and symptoms of someone experiencing a heart attack:

- Chest pain that doesn't go away after 3-5 minutes or chest pain that comes and goes. The person may experience tightness or pressure in the chest, arm, shoulder, jaw, or stomach

- Shortness of breath, difficulty breathing, or fast breathing

- Pale ashen skin

- Dizziness

- Profuse sweating

- Feeling lightheaded

SIGNS OF A HEART ATTACK IN WOMEN

Women often experience additional signs of a heart attack:

- Back pain

- Nausea and vomiting

- Shortness of breath

- Sudden fatigue

Signs of Heart Attack

Symptoms Every Women Should Know and Pay Attention to

Nausea or
vomiting

Shortness
of breath

Pain in arm,
upper back,
neck jaw, or
stomach

Fainting

Breaking out
in a cold sweat

Dizziness or
lightheadedness

Discomfort or pressure
in center of the chest

Paleness or
dummy skin

Inability to sleep

Unusual fatigue

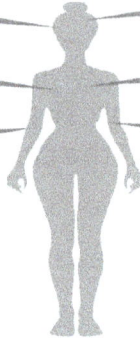

CARE FOR A HEART ATTACK

CPR can prevent further damage to the heart. However, the person will need professional medical care as soon as possible. Call 911 immediately if you suspect the person is experiencing a heart attack.

If the person is conscious:

- Ask if they want you to call 911 and proceed if this is what they want

- Have the person sit as comfortably as possible

- Monitor the person until help arrives

If the person is NOT conscious, you will need to perform CPR.

GIVING CPR

CPR stands for **cardiopulmonary resuscitation**. It is a combination of chest compressions and rescue breaths. Giving CPR helps take over the work of the heart and the lungs while waiting for professional care. Understand that CPR only provides a third of the normal blood to the brain. For that reason, in addition to giving CPR, using an AED gives the person a better chance of survival.

Every minute the person is not receiving care reduces the chance of survival by 10%. Knowing what to do and calling 911 right away is critical.

WHEN AND HOW TO GIVE CPR (ADULTS)

Checking the Person for Responsiveness:
Tap the shoulder and ask:" Are you ok?" If there is no answer,

- Call 911

- Open the airways to check for breathing by performing the ***Head-tilt Chin-lift*** technique

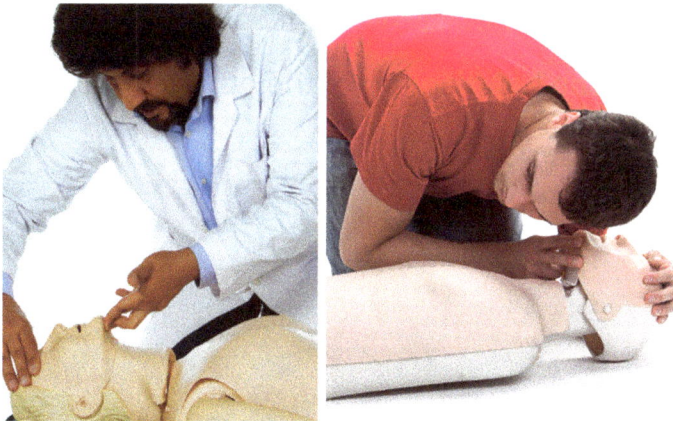

Head-tilt – Chin-lift technique: Look, listen, feel for breathing.

- Determine if the person is still breathing by looking, listening, and feeling for breathing: place your ear close to the nose and mouth. In adults and children, hold the head tilted backward. At the same time, check for a sign of breath (is the chest moving). Only perform CPR if the person is not breathing.

- When performing CPR, move the person to a hard surface; providing CPR on a soft surface is ineffective. Perform 30 chest compressions followed by two rescue breaths, optionally. If you cannot give rescue breaths, give chest compressions continuously.

- CPR is performed in a series of compressions and breaths to keep blood circulating until more advanced medical personnel arrive and take over. Although CPR is only 35% effective in restarting the heart, it mainly keeps blood circulating long enough until the paramedic arrives.

GIVING CPR TO AN ADULT OR CHILD

- Give 30 chest compressions at least two inches deep in adults and about 2 inches deep in children

- Place one hand on top of the other in the center of the chest

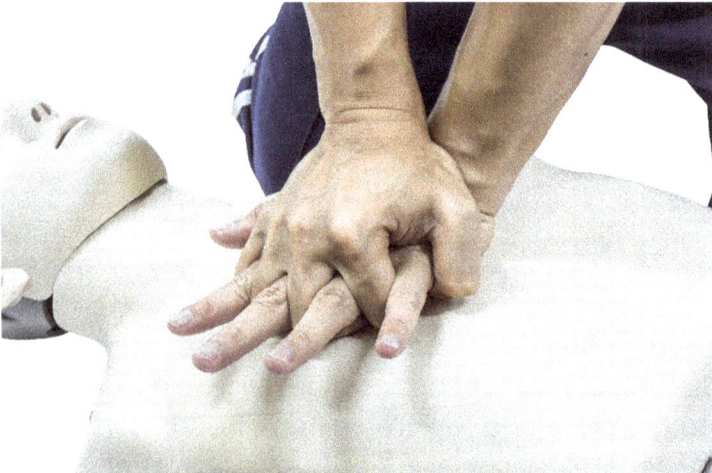

- Stand on your knees with your shoulders stacked directly above your hands

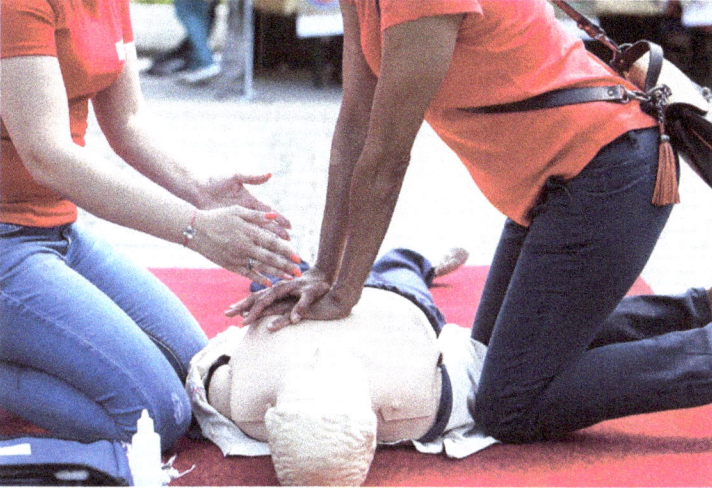

- Give 30 chest compressions at a rate of 100-120 com-pressions per minute

- Give two rescue breaths (optional):

  o Perform the head-tilt chin-lift technique to open the airways,

  o Pinch the person's nose

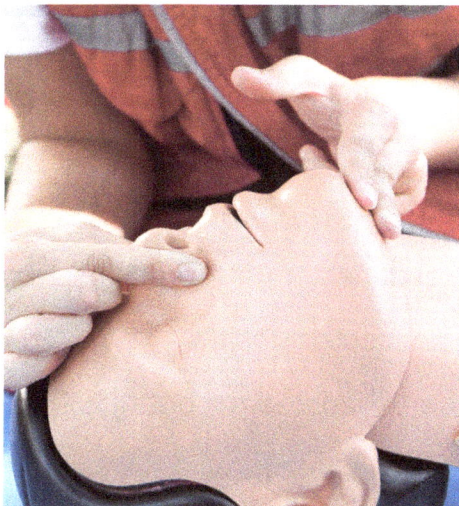

- If you have a breathing barrier, place it over the person's mouth

- Seal your mouth around the person's mouth and blow for about one second, checking that the chest rises. If the chest does not rise, tilt the head back. If the breath doesn't get through, an object might be blocking the airways.

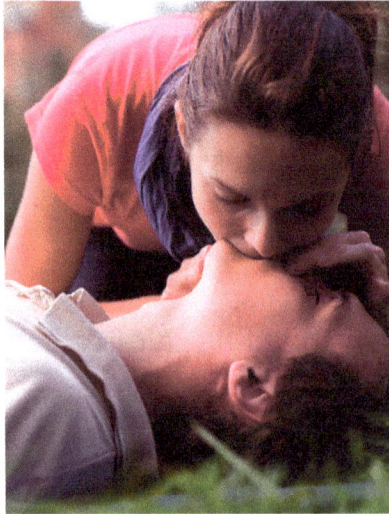

Rescue breath

Continue giving sets of 30 chest compressions and two rescue breaths until

- The person starts breathing again

- Someone qualified or better qualified than you take over

- The scene becomes unsafe

- You are too exhausted to continue

- Your environment is becoming unsafe

- An AED is available to use

WHEN AND HOW TO GIVE CPR (CHILD OR INFANT)

Giving CPR to children and infants is similar to performing CPR on adults. The chart below shows the difference.

	ADULT	CHILD	INFANT
HAND POSITION	2 Hands in the center of the chest	2 Hands in the center of the chest	2-3 fingers in the center of the chest
CHEST COMPRESSION	At least 2 inches deep	About 2 inches deep	About 1.5 inches deep
RESCUE BREATHS	2	2	2
CYCLES	30 chest compressions followed by two breaths	30 chest compressions followed by two breaths	30 chest compressions followed by two breaths
RATE	100 compressions per minute	100 compressions per minute	100 compressions per minute

If you can access an AED (automated electrical defibrillator), use it immediately.

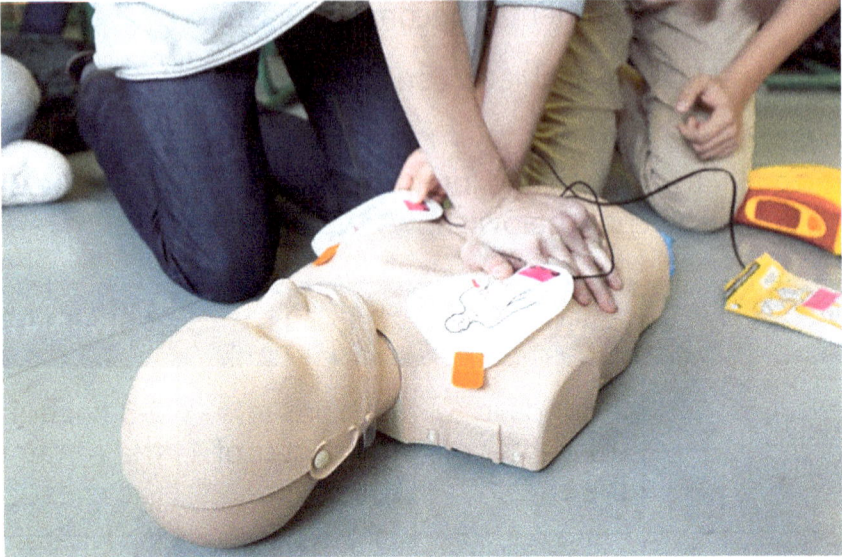

Mannequin with AED pads on the chest

PERFORMING CPR ON AN INFANT

- Do not perform CPR if the infant is breathing. Start by checking for consciousness: flick the bottom of the infant's foot and shout their name if you know it

- If the infant does not react, check for breathing by placing your ear close to the infant's airways and checking for the chest to rise. Do not tilt the head back because their necks are very fragile

- If there are no signs of breathing, place the infant on a firm surface and begin CPR

- Give 30 chest compressions:

  o Place one hand on the infant's forehead

  o Use two or three fingers to give chest compressions 1½ inches deep in the center of the chest, just below the nipple line

  o Perform 100-120 compressions per minute

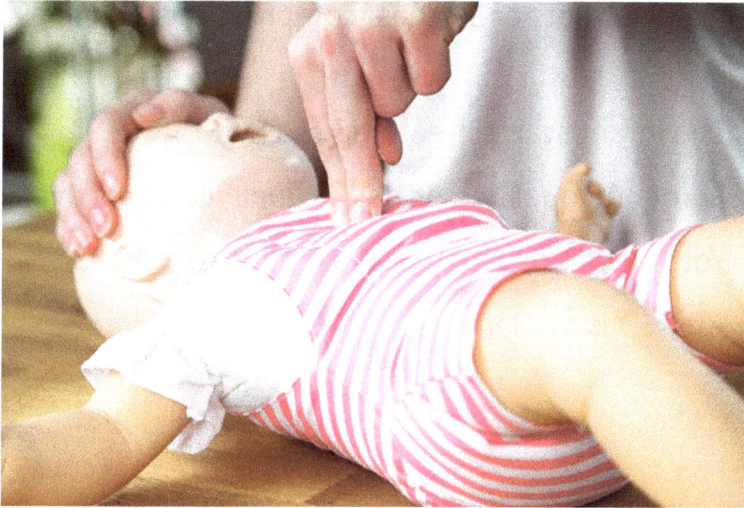

Chest compressions, infant

o   Give two rescue breaths (optional). First, use a breathing barrier, if you have one, to cover the infant's mouth and nose.

o   Make a seal using your mouth over the infant's mouth and nose

o   Blow into their mouth for about one second, checking that their chest rises

o   Repeat with a second rescue breath

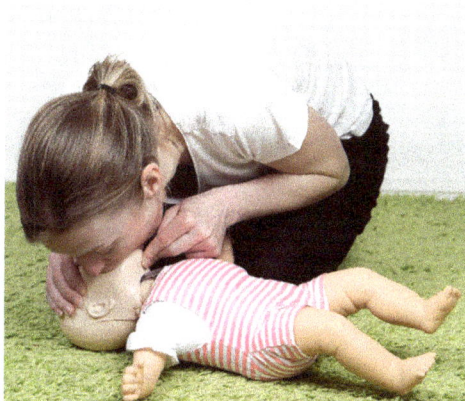

Continue giving sets of 30 chest compressions and two rescue breaths until

- The infant starts breathing again
- Someone qualified or better qualified takes over
- You are too exhausted to continue
- An AED is available

9

HANDLING BREATHNG EMERGENCIES

INTRODUCTION

This chapter will equip you with the basic breathing rescue technique to help someone experiencing a breathing emergency due to choking or asthma.

LEARNING OBJECTIVES

By the end of this chapter, you will know how to:

- Caring for breathing emergencies in a conscious adult or child who is choking

- Caring for breathing emergencies in a conscious infant

BREATHING EMERGENCIES

Choking is a very common breathing emergency, especially in older adults and young children. If the airways are completely blocked, the person will not be able to speak, cough, cry, or breathe and will soon collapse and become unconscious. Some signs the person does not have enough oxygen include the person's face turning bluish. In this situation, call 911 before giving care.

CARE FOR CHOKING – ADULTS AND CHILDREN

- Obtain consent: always ask the person if they need your help

- Encourage the person to keep coughing to help dislodge the object or food

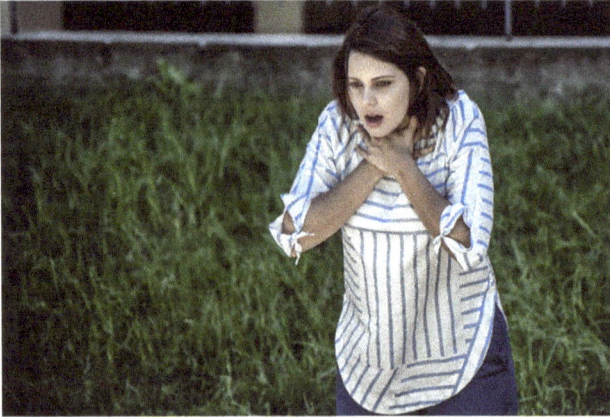

Universal signal for choking

- Ask the person if they want you to call 911

- Stand next to the person, facing toward their hips, with one foot in front of the person and one foot behind the person

- Slide your arm under the person's armpit and across the chest for support

- Using the heel of your hand, proceed with five back blows behind the shoulder blades. The back blows are designed to help dislodge the object blocking the airways

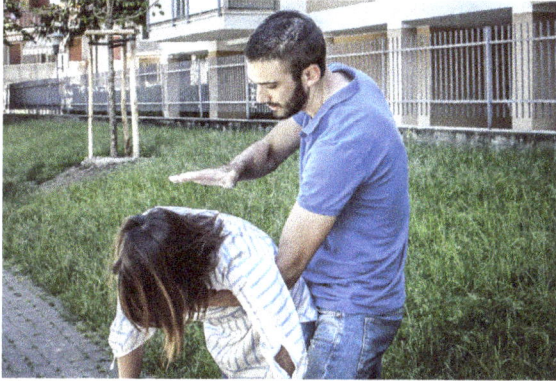

Back blows

- If the person is still choking after five back blows, con- tinue with five abdominal thrusts. First, make a fist and wrap it with the palm of your other hand. Stand behind the person, and place your fist above the person's navel.

- With a child, get on your knees behind the child. The abdominal thrusts create pressure that helps force the blocked object out of the airways.

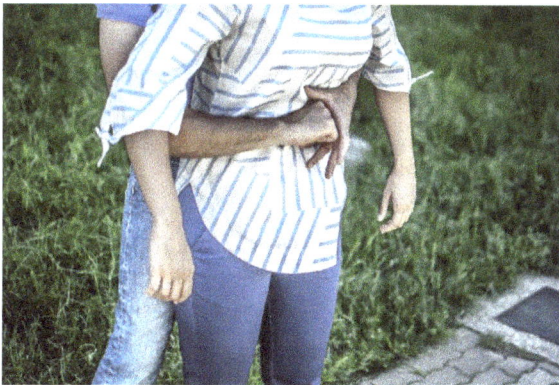

Abdominal Thrust

- Continue alternating with five back blows and five ab- dominal thrusts until the person stops choking, the food or object blocking the airways is expelled, or the person loses consciousness.

If the person becomes unresponsive, gently lower them to the floor and begin modified CPR, starting with chest compressions. After each set of compressions and before attempting rescue breaths, open the person's mouth, look for the object, and remove it if you see it. Never put your finger in the person's mouth unless you see the object.

If You Are Alone
If you are choking and are alone, you can give yourself abdominal thrusts using your fist. The other option is to lean over the back of a chair or a railing to dislodge the object.

If the Person Is Pregnant
If you are pregnant, give the person chest thrusts instead of abdominal thrusts.

CARE FOR CONSCIOUS CHOKING INFANTS

When an infant is conscious but unable to breathe, place the infant on your forearm and perform five back blows and five abdominal thrusts using two fingers.

- Cradle the infant's face and position it down on your forearm. Sit down and rest your forearm on your thigh for support, ensuring the hips are higher than the shoulders. This will help dislodge the object or food blocking the airways. Support the infant's jaw with your fingers. Give five back blows between the shoulder blades with the palm of your hand.

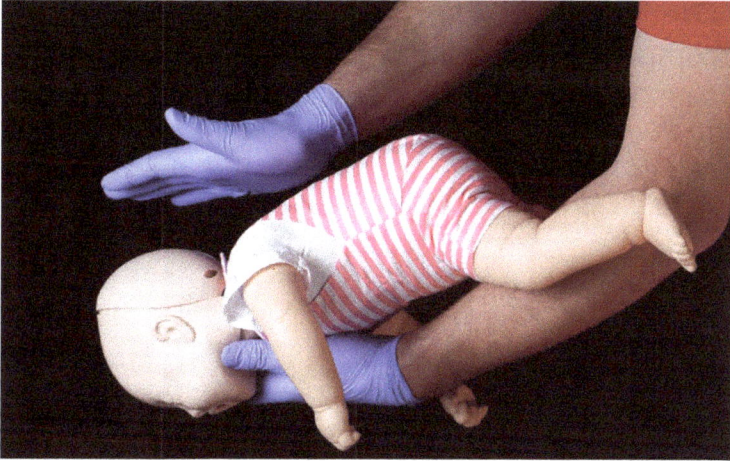

Back blows in infants

- If the infant is still choking, turn them over onto your other arm so that they face up.

- Place two fingers in the center of the chest and perform five abdominal chest compressions.

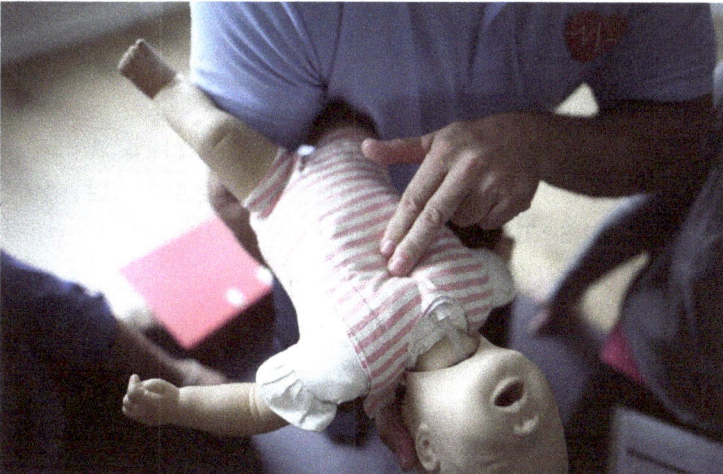

Abdominal thrust on infant

- Continue the cycle of five back blows with five chest compressions until the infant starts breathing or loses consciousness. If the infant is unconscious, begin CPR.

PREVENTING BREATHING EMERGENCIES IN CHILDREN AND INFANTS

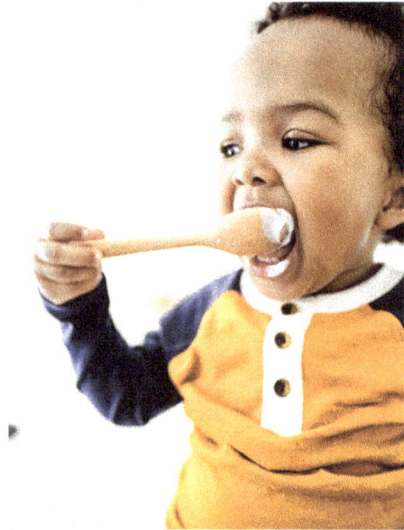

You can take steps to reduce the risks of choking in infants. Children should be supervised when eating and playing. Ensure children remain seated when they eat. Do not feed the following food to children:

- Popcorn
- Grapes
- Chewing gum
- Hard or gooey candy

When giving toys to children, ensure they are age-appropriate by reading the fine print on the back of the packages. Supervise young children at all times when playing with toys.

Be especially careful with the following objects:

- Marbles

- Buttons

- Coins

- Batteries

- Safety pins

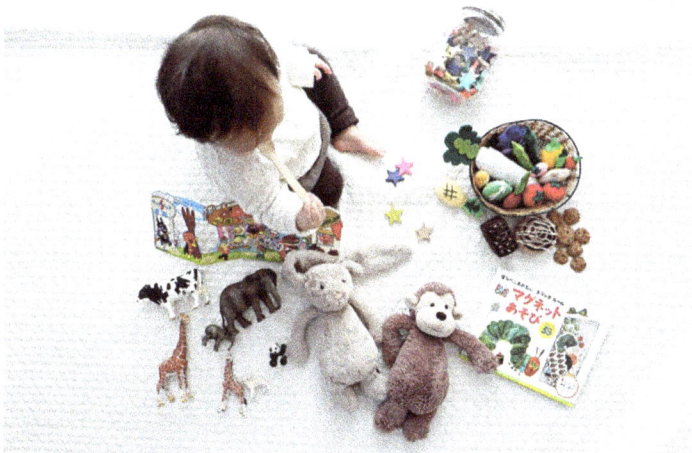

Child playing with toys.

CHAPTER 10

MASTERING SPRAINS AND STRAINS

INTRODUCTION

In uncertain times, when access to medical care is delayed, you must be able to care for yourself or your loved ones without any delay. Common accidents, such as sprains and strains, should be addressed immediately to avoid further tissue damage.

LEARNING OBJECTIVES

In this chapter, you will learn how to:

- Provide first aid care to sprains and strains

- Provide relief for minor sprains and strains

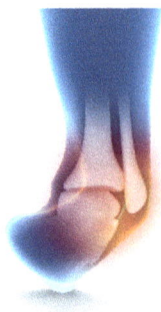

Moderate sprains involve the tearing of some of the ligaments of a joint. This can happen after a fall on an uneven surface, for example. The pain is severe enough to make the person fall or stop all movement at the joint. Swelling and discoloration are common.

STRAINS

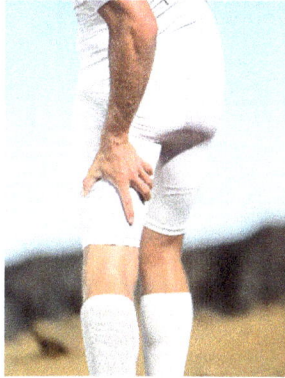

A strain or pull refers to a muscle or muscle group that has been overstretched or torn. It can result from a fall, overexertion while working out, misusing muscles, an accident, or lifting a load that is too heavy.

Like sprains, strains can be very painful, especially in the back, neck, or thigh muscles.

SIGNS AND SYMPTOMS OF MUSCULAR SKELETAL INJURIES
The signs and symptoms of these injuries are often very similar, which may make it difficult to determine one injury from the other. The signs and symptoms include:

- Pain, discomfort
- Swelling

- Discoloration, bruising

- Numbness or tingling

- Deformity, bone sticking out

- Inability to use a body part

- Snapping sound

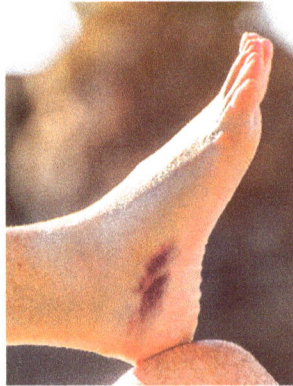

CARE FOR MUSCULOSKELETAL INJURIES

The care for both sprain and strain injuries involves using a technique called **RICE** (**R**est, **I**mmobilize, **C**old, **E**levate)

RICE TECHNIQUE

Rest
Rest is the most important thing to do when you first get injured. Rest will prevent further damage to the injured joint or limb and allow the body to start healing.

Immobilize
In the next chapter, you will learn how to splint an injured limb. **If you are waiting for an ambulance, do not immobilize the limb.**

Cold
Cold lessens the pain and reduces swelling and bleeding.

Make an ice pack by filling a plastic bag with water and ice or using a bag of frozen vegetables. Do not place the ice pack directly on the skin, as this could burn it. Instead, place gauze, a paper towel, or cloth between the ice pack and the skin.

Keep the icepack on the injured limb for 20 minutes, then remove it for 20 minutes. Repeat the cycle of 20 minutes on and 20 minutes off throughout the day.

Elevate
Elevating the injured limb reduces swelling and prevents blood from pooling towards the injury. Only move an injured part if it does not cause further pain.

The **RICE** technique is the first step after a non-severe injury. The second step is to follow up with a medical doctor immediately.

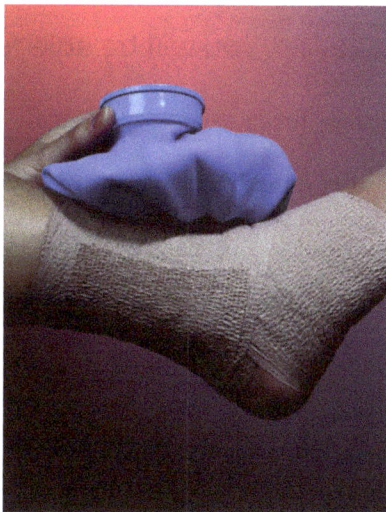

SPLINTING:

ESSENTIAL TECHNIQUES TO SECURE INJURIES

INTRODUCTION

This chapter outlines the techniques for splinting an injured body part using improvised items available at the time of injury. Splinting is the process of immobilizing a limb, which helps support the injured area and reduce pain.

LEARNING OBJECTIVES

After reading this chapter, you will be able to:

- Stabilize injured limb
- Use improvised material to create a sling

GENERAL RULES FOR SPLINTING

- Only splint an injured area if it does not cause more harm or pain
- Keep the limb in the position found; do not try to straighten the limb
- Splint above and below the injury
- Look at the non-injured extremity for circulation. Check the color, temperature, and sensation. Compare both

limbs before and after splinting to make sure it is not too tight

- Elevate the injured area if it does not cause more pain

TYPES OF SPLINTS

SOFT SPLINT

Soft splints are made of cloth, towels, blankets, and pillows and can be used with slings and binders. *A sling and Binder is a specific type of splint that uses a triangular cloth to support and immobilize the shoulder, arm, and elbow. Binders are* fabric used to immobilize an injured arm against the body to provide more support and reduce pain. Binders can be used independently or with a binder to support the injured area.

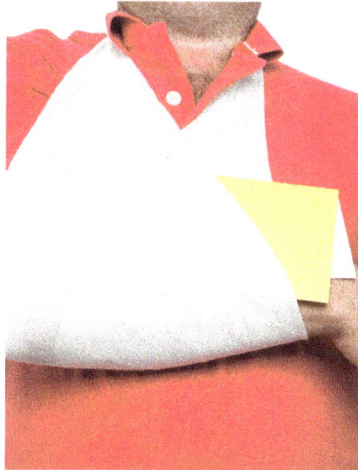

Soft Splint

RIGID SPLINT

A rigid splint is made of rigid materials such as cardboard, magazines, or any rigid object that is available, such as a spoon, plastic, wood, or a ruler.

STEPS FOR SPLINTING

- Gather material around the house, such as rolled-up newspaper, cardboard, rulers, or a rigid board.

- Pad the splinting device with a cloth or soft material to prevent skin discomfort or injury

- Keep the limb in the position found; do not attempt to straighten the limb

- Place the rigid splint underneath and alongside the injured limb. Ensure the splint extends beyond the injury on both sides of the injury

- Secure the splint using a scarf, pillowcase, or sweater underneath the rigid splint and attach the cloth behind the neck.

ANATOMICAL SPLINT

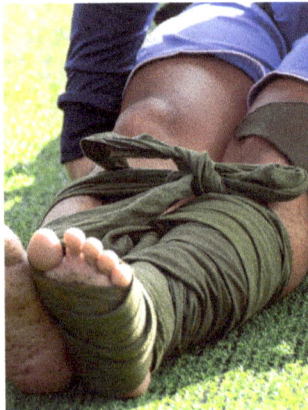

Anatomical Splint

An anatomical splint uses a non-injured body part to support the injured limb. For example, you can splint an injured finger against the rest of the fingers or an injured leg against the non-injured leg. After splinting, check for circulation in the extremities. Check the skin color, warmth, and tingling sensations.

It can be challenging to determine the nature and severity of an injury. For that reason, assume that it is serious. When splinting, focus on providing support and minimizing pain with whatever material you have available. You should not splint an injured limb if an ambulance is on its way.

Emergency First Aid Kit
Organize your bag in compartments that are labeled and dated. Regularly updates expired medicine

- Medical tape
- Nitrile gloves
- Tweezers
- Scissors
- Isopropyl Alcohol, Peroxide
- Saline eye drops
- Irrigation syringe
- Rolled gauze and gauze pads
- Band-Aids
- Pressure dressing
- Moleskin
- Styptic powder
- Antibiotic ointment
- Tourniquests
- Splints
- Pain relievers
- Antihistamines

o   Antacids

o   Prescriptions

o   Thermometer

o   Nail clippers

ESSENTIAL SANITERAY SUPPLIES

You saw in these chapters that prevention goes a long way. You can stockpile enough supplies to last a long time and replace it regularly as it is being used. Keep a log of how much is left, with the date.

o   Toilet paper

o   Baby wipes

o   Soap and hand sanitizer

o   Toothpaste and dental floss

o   Nail clippers and files

o   Razors

o   Deodorant

o   Disposable gloves

o   Masks

o   Feminine hygiene products

o   Garbage bags

o   Diapers

o   Quicklime

o   Insect repellents

o   Bleech

CONCLUSION

Expect the best, plan for the worst, and prepare to be surprised

–Denis Waitley

A sudden loss of power can feel like a seismic shift in our daily lives. The conveniences we've grown accustomed to—hot showers, refrigerated food, and the simple act of flushing a toilet—can vanish overnight. So, how do we best survive without electricity? Where do essential supplies come from when stores are empty? Most importantly, how should basic needs like clean water be met?

If questions like these plagued you in the past, you can now rest at ease. You now have a guide on how to prepare and act during a grid-down crisis. With this knowledge, you can rest easy knowing that you're prepped up for what might hit you. So, go down to the store while it's open, explore the options to prepare your stock-up supplies, and start preparing for a grid-down today!

ESSENTIAL GRID-DOWN SURVIVAL CHECKLISTS

ESSENTIAL GRID-DOWN CHECKLIST
FAMILY EVACUATION BAG

PREPARE FOR EMERGENCIES WITH THIS ESSENTIAL EVACUATION GO-BAG CHECKLIST. ENSURE YOUR BAG IS LIGHTWEIGHT, DURABLE, AND EASY TO CARRY.

PERSONAL ESSENTIALS

- ◯ Identification (ID, passports, birth certificates)
- ◯ Cash (small denominations)
- ◯ Emergency contact list (written down)
- ◯ Map of your local area

CLOTHING

- ◯ Weather-appropriate clothing (2-3 sets)
- ◯ Sturdy shoes
- ◯ Warm hat and gloves (if applicable)
- ◯ Rain poncho

FOOD AND WATER

- ◯ Non-perishable snacks (energy bars, trail mix)
- ◯ Water bottles or collapsible containers
- ◯ Water purification tablets or filter
- ◯ Manual can opener

HEALTH AND HYGIENE

- ◯ First aid kit (bandages, antiseptic, pain relievers)
- ◯ Prescription medications (7-day supply)
- ◯ Hand sanitizer and wet wipes
- ◯ Toothbrush, toothpaste, and travel soap

TOOLS AND SAFETY GEAR

- ◯ Flashlight (with extra batteries or hand-crank)
- ◯ Multi-tool or pocketknife
- ◯ Whistle (for signaling)
- ◯ Extra batteries, Duct tape, scissors,

ESSENTIAL GRID-DOWN CHECKLIST
FAMILY EVACUATION BAG

PREPARE FOR EMERGENCIES WITH THIS ESSENTIAL EVACUATION GO-BAG CHECKLIST. ENSURE YOUR BAG IS LIGHTWEIGHT, DURABLE, AND EASY TO CARRY.

COMMUNICATION AND NAVIGATION

- Portable phone charger (solar-powered or battery pack)
- Battery-powered or hand-crank radio
- Compass

SHELTER AND COMFORT

- Emergency blanket
- Compact sleeping bag or bivvy sack
- Lightweight tent or tarp

MISCELLANEOUS

- Copies of important documents (sealed in waterproof bags)
- Small notebook and pen
- Spare keys (home and car)

FOR FAMILIES WITH CHILDREN OR PETS

- Baby supplies (diapers, formula, baby food)
- Pet supplies (food, leash, carrier)

KEEP YOUR GO-BAG UPDATED EVERY SIX MONTHS AND STORE IT IN AN EASILY ACCESSIBLE LOCATION.

DOWNLOAD AND PRINT THIS CHECKLIST TO STAY PREPARED!

ESSENTIAL GRID-DOWN CHECKLIST
INFANT EVACUATION BAG

WHEN EVACUATING WITH AN INFANT, PREPARATION IS CRUCIAL. PACK THESE ESSENTIALS TO ENSURE YOUR BABY'S NEEDS ARE MET IN ANY EMERGENCY.

FEEDING ESSENTIALS

- ◯ Formula (enough for 3-5 days)
- ◯ Pre-filled bottles or collapsible bottles
- ◯ Breast pump (manual or battery-powered)
- ◯ Baby food (ready-to-eat jars/pouches)
- ◯ Bibs and burp cloths

CLOTHING AND WARMTH

- ◯ Onesies or bodysuits (5-7)
- ◯ Warm clothes (seasonal-appropriate)
- ◯ Hats and socks
- ◯ Swaddle blankets or sleep sacks

DIAPERING AND HYGIENE

- ◯ Diapers (supply for 3-5 days)
- ◯ Wipes (unscented)
- ◯ Diaper cream
- ◯ Changing pad
- ◯ Plastic bags (for soiled items)

HEALTH AND COMFORT

- ◯ Infant first aid kit (include baby thermometer, saline drops)
- ◯ Pacifiers (extras in case one gets lost)
- ◯ Teething toys or remedies
- ◯ Favorite blanket or lovey for comfort

ESSENTIAL GRID-DOWN CHECKLIST
INFANT EVACUATION BAG

WHEN EVACUATING WITH AN INFANT, PREPARATION IS CRUCIAL. PACK THESE ESSENTIALS TO ENSURE YOUR BABY'S NEEDS ARE MET IN ANY EMERGENCY.

SLEEPING AND CARRYING

○ Portable crib or travel bassinet (if space allows)
○ Baby carrier or sling

EMERGENCY SUPPLIES

○ Emergency contact list
○ Copies of baby's medical records and immunization card
○ Photo ID of the baby (if available)
○ Lightweight tarp or waterproof mat for shelter

EXTRAS FOR PEACE OF MIND

○ Spare phone charger (battery pack or solar-powered)
○ Small toys or books to soothe and entertain

ENSURE YOUR INFANT GO-BAG IS CHECKED AND REFRESHED EVERY 3-6 MONTHS TO ACCOMMODATE GROWING NEEDS.

DOWNLOAD AND PRINT THIS CHECKLIST TO STAY PREPARED!

ESSENTIAL GRID-DOWN CHECKLIST
PET EVACUATION BAG

ENSURE YOUR FURRY COMPANIONS ARE SAFE AND COMFORTABLE DURING EMERGENCIES WITH THIS ESSENTIAL PET GO-BAG CHECKLIST.

FOOD AND WATER

- ◯ Pet food (3-5 day supply, dry or wet)
- ◯ Collapsible food and water bowls
- ◯ Water bottles or portable containers
- ◯ Treats

HYGIENE AND CLEAN-UP

- ◯ Waste bags for cleanup
- ◯ Disposable litter box and litter (for cats)
- ◯ Pet-safe wipes for cleaning
- ◯ Towels (small and lightweight)

HEALTH AND SAFETY

- ◯ Pet first aid kit (include bandages, antiseptic, tweezers)
- ◯ Current medications (5-7 day supply)
- ◯ Vaccination records and medical history (in a waterproof bag)
- ◯ Flea/tick prevention
- ◯ Muzzle (if needed for safety)

IDENTIFICATION

- ◯ Current photo of your pet
- ◯ Microchip ID number
- ◯ Tags with updated contact information
- ◯ Leash and collar or harness

ESSENTIAL GRID-DOWN CHECKLIST
PET EVACUATION BAG

ENSURE YOUR FURRY COMPANIONS ARE SAFE AND COMFORTABLE DURING EMERGENCIES WITH THIS ESSENTIAL PET GO-BAG CHECKLIST.

COMFORT ITEMS

- ○ Favorite toy or chew item
- ○ Blanket or familiar bedding

TRANSPORT AND SHELTER

- ○ Pet carrier or crate (labeled with pet's name and your contact info)
- ○ Tarp or ground cover (for outdoor shelter)

EMERGENCY SUPPLIES

- ○ List of nearby pet-friendly shelters and emergency contacts
- ○ Extra set of your pet's tags and ID
- ○ Spare leash or harness

CHECK AND UPDATE YOUR PET'S GO-BAG REGULARLY TO ENSURE IT MEETS THEIR NEEDS.

DOWNLOAD AND PRINT THIS CHECKLIST TO STAY PREPARED!

ESSENTIAL GRID-DOWN CHECKLIST
FIRST AID BAG

BE READY TO HANDLE MEDICAL EMERGENCIES DURING A GRID-DOWN SITUATION WITH THIS COMPREHENSIVE FIRST AID KIT CHECKLIST

BASIC SUPPLIES

- Adhesive bandages (assorted sizes)
- Sterile gauze pads (various sizes)
- Medical adhesive tape
- Elastic bandages (ACE wraps)
- Triangular bandage (for slings or support)
- Butterfly closures

ANTISEPTICS AND CLEANING SUPPLIES

- Antiseptic wipes
- Hydrogen peroxide or isopropyl alcohol
- Antibiotic ointment (e.g., Neosporin)
- Saline solution (for wound irrigation)

PAIN RELIEF AND MEDICATIONS

- Pain relievers (ibuprofen, acetaminophen)
- Antihistamines (for allergies, e.g., Benadryl)
- Anti-diarrheal medication
- Antacids
- Prescription medications (7-day supply)
- Personal medications (labeled and in waterproof containers)

TOOLS AND INSTRUMENTS

- Scissors (medical-grade)
- Tweezers (for splinters, debris)
- Thermometer (digital or manual)
- Safety pins (assorted sizes)
- Splinting materials (foldable or inflatable)
- Flashlight with extra batteries or hand-crank

ESSENTIAL GRID-DOWN CHECKLIST
FIRST AID BAG

BE READY TO HANDLE MEDICAL EMERGENCIES DURING A GRID-DOWN SITUATION WITH THIS COMPREHENSIVE FIRST AID KIT CHECKLIST

DRESSINGS AND WOUND CARE

- ○ Non-stick sterile pads
- ○ Wound closure strips (e.g., Steri-Strips)
- ○ Burn cream or gel
- ○ Petroleum jelly (for skin protection)
- ○ Disposable gloves (non-latex preferred)

HYGIENE AND PROTECTIVE GEAR

- ○ Face masks (N95 or surgical)
- ○ Hand sanitizer
- ○ Soap or antiseptic hand wash
- ○ Waste bags for medical disposal

ADDITIONAL EMERGENCY ITEMS

- ○ CPR mask or face shield
- ○ Emergency blanket (foil-type)
- ○ Cold packs (instant)
- ○ Hot packs (chemical or reusable)
- ○ Cotton balls and swabs

INSTRUCTIONS AND DOCUMENTATION

- ○ First aid manual or quick reference guide
- ○ Personal medical history forms for family members

SPECIALIZED ITEMS

- ○ EpiPen (if prescribed for severe allergies)
- ○ Snake bite kit (if in a high-risk area)
- ○ Eye wash solution (or eye dropper)
- ○ Splinter removers

REFERENCES

Ajmera, R. (2020, January 15). *Does water expire?* Healthline. https://www.healthline.com/nutrition/does-water-expire

Bauer, B. A. (2023, March 24). *What is BPA, and what are the concerns about BPA?* Mayo Clinic. https://www.mayoclinic.org/healthy-lifestyle/nutrition-and-healthy-eating/expert-answers/bpa/faq-20058331

Bodnar, P. (2021, June 22). *How to sanitize water bottles with bleach.* FarOut. https://faroutguides.com/how-to-sanitize-water-bottles-with-bleach/

Boil water advisory. (2023, April 13). CDC.

Burnside, T., & Salahieh, N. (2024, February 4). More than 800,000 without power in California as intense atmospheric river brings threat of mudslides and flooding. *CNN.* https://edition.cnn.com/2024/02/04/us/california-atmospheric-river-flooding/index.html

Earthquakes and seismic protection for Japanese nuclear power plants. (2017, May 31). World Nuclear Association. https://world-nuclear.org/information-library/appendices/earthquakes-and-seismic-protection-for-japanes-(1)

Garvey, M. (2018, June 19). *Checklist: Making a first aid kit for baby.* TheBUMP. https://www.thebump.com/a/making-a-first-aid-kit-for-baby

The *impact of power outages.* (n.d.). Pinkerton. https://pinkerton.com/our-insights/blog/the-impact-of-power-outages

Lafleur, J. (2018, July 18). *Expect the best, plan for the worst, and prepare to be surprised.* Lehigh University. https://engineering.lehigh.edu/news/article/%E2%80%9Cexpect-best-plan-worst-and-prepare-be-surprised%E2%80%9Ds

O'Neill, P. H. (2022, April 12). *Russian hackers tried to bring down Ukraine's power grid to help the invasion.* MIT Technology Review. https://www.technologyreview.com/2022/04/12/1049586/russian-hackers-tried-to-bring-down-ukraines-power-grid-to-help-the-invasion/

Power grid cyberattack in Ukraine (2015). (n.d.). Cyber Law Toolkit. https://cyberlaw.ccdcoe.org/wiki/Power_grid_cyberattack_in_Ukraine_(2015)

Quadir, R. (2012, July 25). *Startling facts you should know about disaster preparedness*. Centers for Disease Control and Prevention. https://blogs.cdc.gov/publichealthmatters/2012/07/startling-facts-you-should-know-about-disaster-preparedness/

Roberts, A. (2023, April 2). *Si vis pacem, para bellum*. Adam's Notebook. https://medium.com/adams-notebook/si-vis-pacem-para-bellum-a5ad331c0e4

Sayner, A. (2021, July 27). *How to build a root cellar: A step by step guide*. GroCycle. https://grocycle.com/how-to-build-a-root-cellar/

10 worst blackouts of the last 50 years. (2015, January 13). Power Technology. https://www.power-technology.com/features/featurethe-10-worst-blackouts-in-the-last-50-years-4486990/?cf-view

Urban survival training, skills, preparation, resources. (n.d.). SBS Training Solutions. https://www.sbstrains.com/urban-survival-training

Warmth and temperature regulation. (2014, August 24). Children's Hospital of Philadelphia. https://www.chop.edu/conditions-diseases/warmth-and-temperature-regulation

Wolf, C. (2024, May 4). *How to survive without electricity*. How to Survive Everything. https://howtosurviveeverything.com/how-to-survive-without-electricity/

IMAGE REFERENCES

Ezvedat. (2024, January 7). *Kettle over campfire* [Image]. Pexels. https://www.pexels.com/photo/kettle-over-campfire-19778250/

Henry, M. (n.d.). *Cute baby girls face close up* [Image]. Shopify. https://www.shopify.com/stock-photos/photos/cute-baby-girls-face-close-up?q=cute+kids

J, M. (2022, March 24). *A sign showing the direction of the evacuation route on the beach* [Image]. Pexels. https://www.pexels.com/photo/a-sign-showing-the-direction-of-the-evacuation-route-on-the-beach-17122126/

Jackson, D. (2016, June 18). *Pickles on glass jars* [Image]. Pexels. https://www.pexels.com/photo/pickles-on-glass-jars-6611594/

Loubier, C. (2019, April 25). *Man soaked in body of water* [Image]. Unsplash. https://unsplash.com/photos/man-soaked-in-body-of-water-gAontQPkqls

Nishizuka. (2012, October 14). *Brown chihuahua* [Image]. Pexels. https://www.pexels.com/photo/brown-chihuahua-485294/

Pham, A. (2017, December 6). *Two person holding fork dipping food on sauce* [Image]. Unsplash. https://unsplash.com/photos/two-person-holding-fork-dipping-food-on-sauce-vo7GGTh6sXM

Partners, S. (n.d.). *Steak and flames on the grill* [Image]. Shopify. https://www.shopify.com/stock-photos/photos/steak-and-flames-on-the-grill?q=grill

Seiler, K. (2019, March). *Firemen performing drill outdoors* [Image]. Unsplash. https://unsplash.com/photos/firemen-performing-drill-outdoors-yvjSFEMWoGk

Zerdzicki, J. (2024, March 26). *Fire alarm* [Image]. Pexels. https://www.pexels.com/photo/fire-alarm-21299748/

www.ingramcontent.com/pod-product-compliance
Lightning Source LLC
Chambersburg PA
CBHW071228290326
41931CB00037B/2452